200
Chest X-ray
Cases

The
London
Press

FOREWORD

Modern medical practice has seen many advances in imaging over the past ten years. Magnetic Resonance Imaging, CT scanning and Ultrasound investigations have all been added to the repertoire of normal practice. However, the humble chest X-ray remains a crucial first line investigation – particularly for acute medical admissions.

Many chest X-rays are requested for a specific purpose e.g. confirmation of pneumonia, but the image may reveal features of previously unsuspected disease of another body system.

Digital storage of X-ray images means that a chest X-ray may be viewed at any computer workstation in your hospital. Clinicians now have the opportunity to view these images without waiting for the X-ray packet to be delivered. This can only be advantageous for the patient if the clinician knows what to look for on the image.

This book takes you through 200 images in a stimulating manner designed to improve your confidence in reporting the humble chest X-ray.

Dr Anthony J FRANCE M.A. M.B. B.Chir. F.R.C.P.Ed
Consultant Physician, Respiratory and Infectious Diseases
Ninewells Hospital and Medical School, Dundee.

ACKNOWLEDGMENT

"We would like to thank Dr William Anderson, Dr Adam Hill, Dr Philip Short, Dr Arun Nair and Dr RP Smith for providing the authors with several of the X-ray images reproduced in this work.

Sincere gratitude towards Dr JH Winter, for reviewing all the incorporated X-ray images and providing us with helpful guidance on clinical interpretation, X-ray reports and the questions set for each CXR case.

Last but not least, many thanks to NHS Tayside's department of Radiology for providing us with most of the x-rays images reproduced within these pages."

Chest X-ray interpretation is an essential skill for clinical medicine, but a skill often neglected in the medical school curriculum and in post-graduate training.

Like so many skills, we learn by "doing" rather than by rote. We would argue that the ability to read a chest x-ray accurately is proportionate to the number of x-rays you have actually seen in a career.

The authors have a colleague with such legendary skill in interpreting the CXR it is said he once diagnosed Tinea Pedis from the chest image! Such skills are not acquired by some magical ability or arcane knowledge, but simply by having seen a particular abnormality before, and knowing its clinical significance.

200 Chest X-rays is therefore unique in allowing you to see 200 of the most important clinical abnormalities on the chest x-ray. Collected from the outpatient clinics and emergency departments on a Scottish hospital, these are not a library of unusual or rare disorders, but a practical guide to what you are going to see during your daily life as a physician- and critically- what to do about it.

We have included "Best of five" format questions with every case to make the book a more enjoyable and an interactive read and hopefully an additional tool to those planning to sit membership exams. Questions will also be given a 1, 2 or 3 star rating where we expect final year medical students and those at foundation training to correctly answer 1 star questions, those at specialty training level to answer 2 star questions and 3 star questions are reserved for those respiratory physicians among us!

We hope you like the book and hope your patients will benefit from the skills you acquire.

Mudher ZH Al-Khairalla
James D Chalmers
Tom C Fardon
August 2009

BEFORE YOU BEGIN...

Before reporting the chest x-ray

Confirm the following:

Patient details, date of the film and x-ray projection (Posterior-Anterior (PA), Anterior-Posterior (AP) and lateral views). PA films usually provide the best technical films for interpretation as the cardiac silhouette is not magnified and the lung fields are not obstructed by the scapulae. Chest x-rays A, B and C illustrate the anatomy. An adequate film is central (the spinus process is equidistant between the ends of each clavicle head), well penetrated (the vertebral bodies are easily identified behind the heart) and adequately inspired (indicated by 6 anterior ribs visible over the lung fields). For each case, we will comment on technical aspects prior to interpreting the film. "Technically adequate" implies central plain film that is well inspired, penetrated and an adequate field of view is captured.

Approach the X-ray systematically. This is important, so that important pathology is not missed. Don't be distracted by the big tumour and miss the shoulder fracture too!

Many systems and acronyms have been promoted, but tend to confuse the issue. The authors approach is simple and is described in the appendix at the end of the book.

ABBREVIATIONS*

UZ = Upper zone

MZ = Mid zone

LZ = Lower zone

R = Right

L = Left

UL = Upper Lobe

ML = Middle Lobe

LL = Lower lobe

CXR = Chest X-ray

* Other abbreviations are highlighted in the text

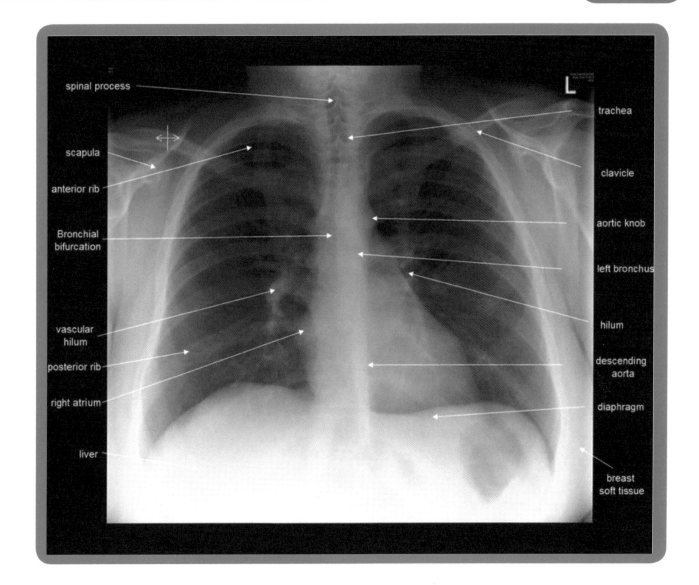

spinal process

trachea

L

scapula

clavicle

anterior rib

aortic knob

Bronchial
bifurcation

left bronchus

vascular
hilum

hilum

posterior rib

descending
aorta

right atrium

diaphragm

liver

breast
soft tissue

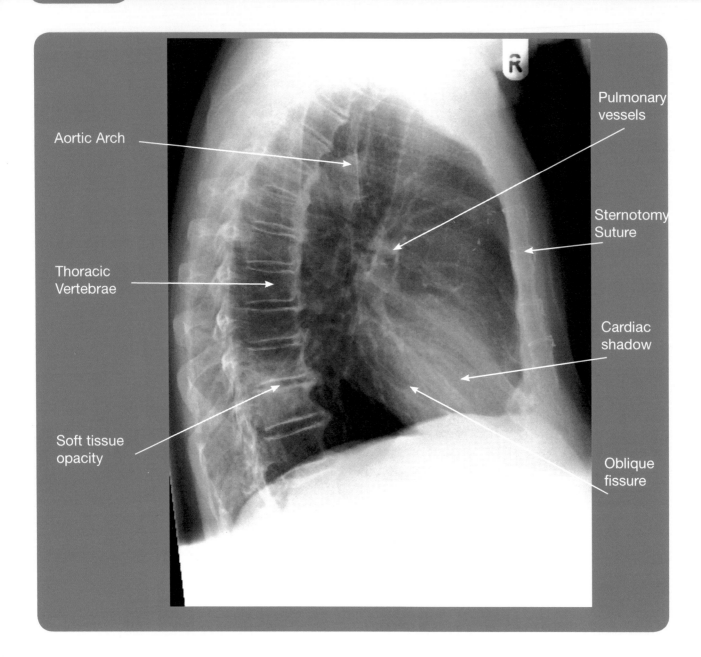

Aortic Arch

Thoracic Vertebrae

Soft tissue opacity

Pulmonary vessels

Sternotomy Suture

Cardiac shadow

Oblique fissure

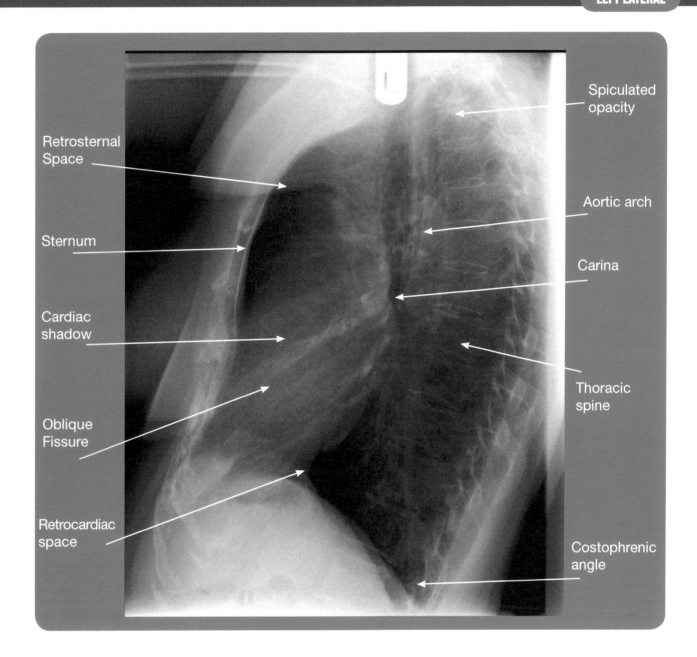

Spiculated opacity

Retrosternal Space

Sternum

Cardiac shadow

Oblique Fissure

Retrocardiac space

Aortic arch

Carina

Thoracic spine

Costophrenic angle

Q **: What is the most likely diagnosis**

1. Pulmonary oedema

2. Right Pulmonary embolism

3. Parapneumonic effusion

4. Malignant Effusion

5. Left lower lobe lung abscess

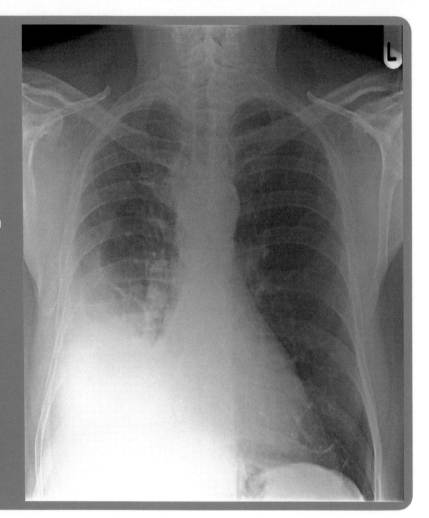

THIS CXR SHOWS

Projection: PA, well centred, under penetrated, adequate field of view.

There is homogenous dense opacification in the right lower zone.

Midline sternotomy sutures in keeping with previous cardiac surgery.

CLINICAL INTERPRETATION

This woman had signs suggestive of a right sided pleural effusion. Clinical suspicion was of simple or complicated parapneumonic effusion, or empyema.

Diagnostic pleural aspiration confirmed thick, cloudy pleural fluid with a pH of < 7.2, confirming complicated parapneumonic effusion.

Treatment was intravenous antibiotics and intercostal pleural drainage with a 12 F drain, flushed 6 hourly with 50 mls of 0.9 % saline.

Answer: 3) Parapneumonic effusion ★

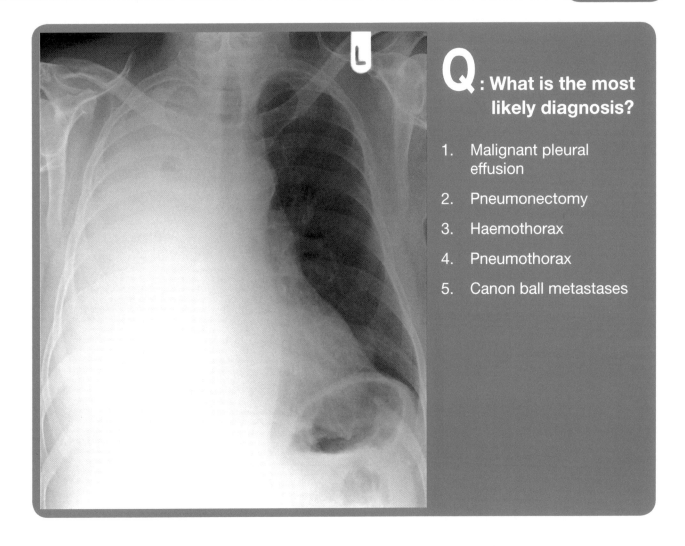

Q: What is the most likely diagnosis?

1. Malignant pleural effusion
2. Pneumonectomy
3. Haemothorax
4. Pneumothorax
5. Canon ball metastases

THIS CXR SHOWS

Projection: PA, well centred, under penetrated, adequate field of view.

Complete white out of the right hemithorax with no mediastinal shift

CLINICAL INTERPRETATION

Causes of complete "white-out" are:

- Pleural effusion (which includes haemothorax)
- Complete Lung Collapse
- Pneumonectomy

Mediastinal shift or its absence will help to differentiate the above causes.

This patient had known renal carcinoma complicated by symptomatic disseminated malignant pleural effusion.

Q : What is the most likely cause for the raised right hemidiaphragm?

1. Liver enlargement
2. Pulmonary embolism
3. Laryngeal nerve palsy
4. RML pneumonia
5. Right lower lobectomy

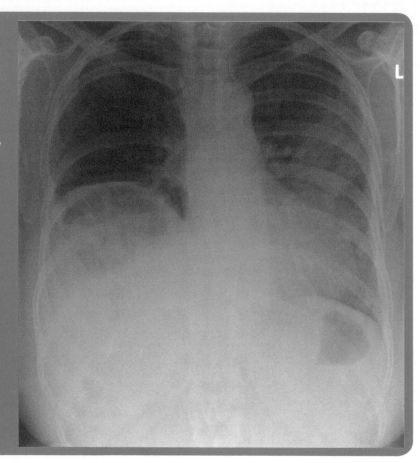

L

THIS CXR SHOWS

Projection: PA, well centred, well penetrated, adequate field of view.

Missing right 5th rib

Elevated right hemidiaphragm secondary to previous right lower lobectomy for tuberculosis many years ago LMZ airspace opacification

CLINICAL INTERPRETATION

This woman has left midzone consolidation; combined with her clinical presentation of cough, fever and raised inflammatory markers the diagnosis is community acquired pneumonia.

The changes at the right base are long standing. It is important to see previous x-rays – without them it is often impossible to differentiate acute from chronic changes.

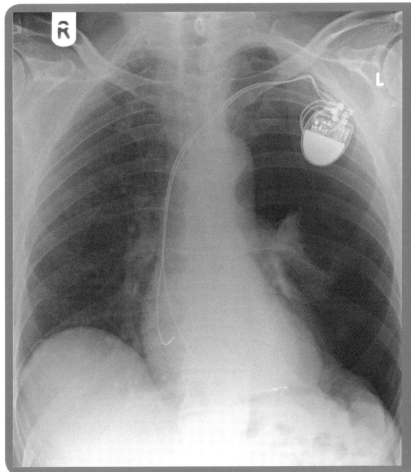

Q : What is the recommended treatment in this case?

1. Observation
2. Intercostal chest drain
3. Diagnostic pleural tap
4. Pacemaker re-insertion
5. Therapeutic aspiration

THIS CXR SHOWS

Projection: PA, well centred, well penetrated, adequate field of view.

Dual chamber pacemaker positioned in the LUZ complete left sided pneumothorax with no mediastinal shift.

The atrial lead is malpositioned.

CLINICAL INTERPRETATION

This is an iatrogenic cause of pneumothorax. Mediastinal shift is a common finding with any pneumothorax, but does not imply tension. Tension pneumothorax is a clinical diagnosis suggested by cardiac compromise in association with pneumothorax. In this case the patient developed ventricular tachycardia and hypotension. Immediate thoracocentesis to relieve the tension was followed by insertion of an intercostal chest drain.

Q: What is the most likely diagnosis?

1. Tuberculosis
2. Non-Hodgkins Lymphoma
3. Histoplasmosis
4. Sarcoidosis
5. Hodgkins lymphoma

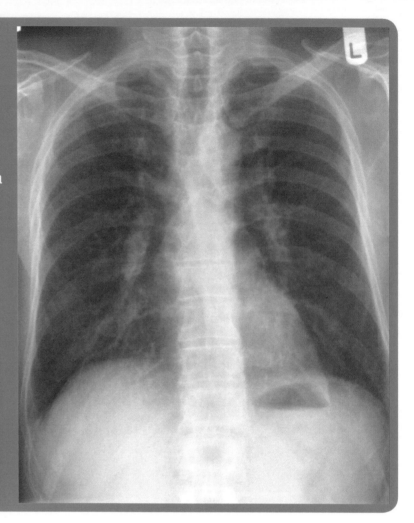

THIS CXR SHOWS

Projection: PA, well centred, well penetrated, adequate field of view.

Bilateral hilar lymphadenopathy with pulmonary nodularity.

CLINICAL INTERPRETATION

The clinical presentation of bilateral hilar lymphadenopathy (BHL) and lower limb lesions suggestive of erythema nodosum (EN) can be explained by the unifying diagnosis of Sarcoidosis. This is more common in Afro-Carribeans. A common subtype of acute sarcoidosis known as Lofgren's syndrome (BHL, EN and arthralgia) typically has a good prognosis. This case is not typical of Lofgren's syndrome in view of the presence of lung nodularity and therefore parenchymal involvement. The main differentials of BHL are tuberculosis and lymphoproliferative disease.

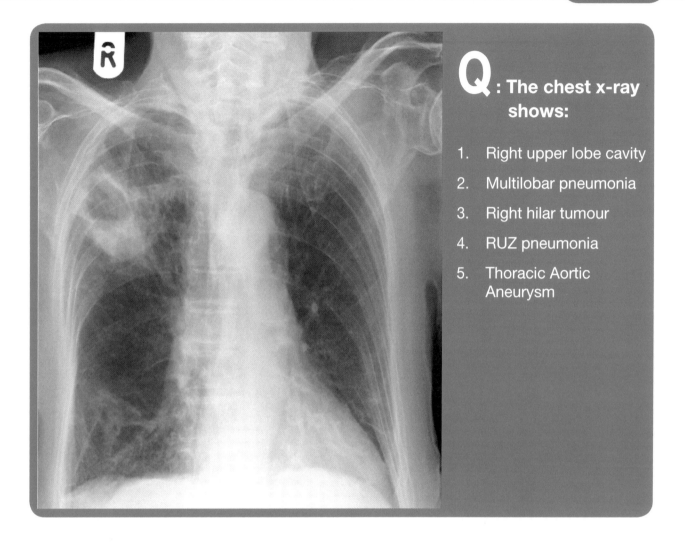

Q: The chest x-ray shows:

1. Right upper lobe cavity
2. Multilobar pneumonia
3. Right hilar tumour
4. RUZ pneumonia
5. Thoracic Aortic Aneurysm

THIS CXR SHOWS

Projection: PA, rotated to the left, well penetrated, adequate field of view.

There is an air-fluid level in the right upper zone, suggestive of a cavity. There is also patchy consolidation in the right lower zone.

CLINICAL INTERPRETATION

A horizontal line on a CXR represents an air-fluid interface. An air-fluid level in a cavity suggests abscess or cavitating tumour. In this case abscess was confirmed on CT scanning of the thorax.

Common causes of cavitating pneumonia are *staphylococcus aureus* and *klebsiella pneumoniae*. *Mycobacterium Tuberculosis* must also be considered.

10% of squamous cell carcinomas cavitate. Cavitation is unusual in other cell types.

CXR 7

This 70 year old woman has a history of rheumatoid arthritis. She presented with breathlessness

Q **: The most likely diagnosis is?:**

1. Pulmonary oedema

2. Eosinophilic pneumonia

3. Nitrofurantoin pneumonitis

4. Acute interstitial pneumonia

5. Usual interstitial pneumonia

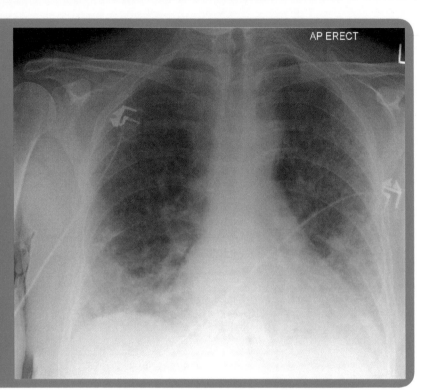

THIS CXR SHOWS

Projection: PA, well centred, adequate penetration, adequate field of view.

There is peripheral opacification with a reticular, interstitial pattern affecting all lobes with a basal predominance.

Leads from a cardiac monitor are noted.

CLINICAL INTERPRETATION

In a patient with rheumatoid arthritis presenting with breathlessness these changes are highly suggestive of rheumatoid associated interstitial lung disease and pulmonary fibrosis.

Pulmonary fibrosis may occur as a complication of sero-positive rheumatoid arthritis or as a complication of treatment with methotrexate. Rheumatoid associated interstitial fibrosis is usually of a usual interstitial pneumonia pattern[1]. Acute interstitial pneumonia is unusual in RA but relatively common in patients with SLE.

[1] Curr Opin Pulm Med. 2006; 12(5):346-53.

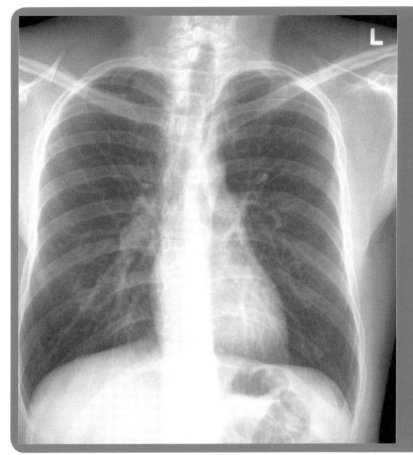

Q: What is the most likely diagnosis?

1. Tuberculosis
2. Pneumocystic Jirovecii pneumonia
3. Normal
4. Pulmonary hypertension
5. HIV seroconversion illness

THIS CXR SHOWS

Projection: PA, slightly rotated to the left, well penetrated, adequate field of view.

Mild scoliosis, otherwise normal CXR!

CLINICAL INTERPRETATION

This is the CXR of one of the authors (Al-Khairalla)! Fortunately there is no cavitating lesion on the film!

However, *Pneumocystic Jirovecii pneumonia* can still present with dry cough and a normal CXR but it was felt that the patient was low risk!

People who go to the hajj are at increased risk of cross infection in view of the millions of people that attend this event annually.

Q: What is the next most appropriate investigation?

1. Sputum cytology
2. Bronchoscopy
3. CT guided lung biopsy
4. Mediastinoscopy
5. Mantoux test

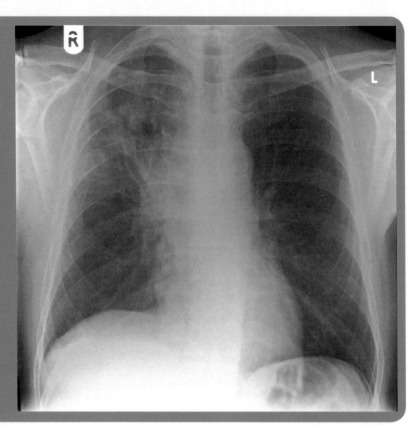

THIS CXR SHOWS

Projection: PA, well centred, well penetrated, adequate field of view.

Dense right hilar opacity extending into the RUZ with volume loss.

CLINICAL INTERPRETATION

Volume loss suggests lobar collapse – this was confirmed at bronchoscopy - this gentleman had non small cell carcinoma completely occluding his right upper lobe bronchus.

In the clinical context of possible malignancy, the chest x-ray guides investigation - centrally placed tumours are more likely to be accessible at bronchoscopy, particularly if causing volume loss. Bronchoscopy rarely yields a diagnosis when the CXR lesion is peripheral.

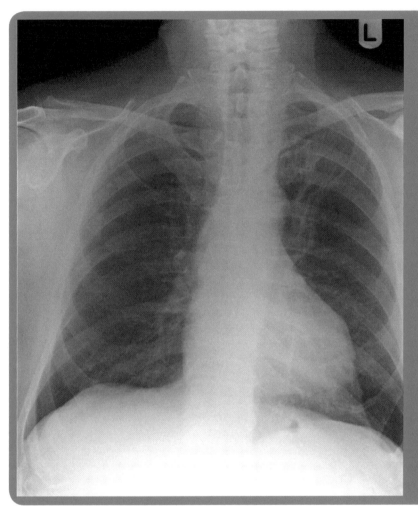

Q: Which of the following is the **least** possible cause of this patients haemoptysis?

1. Tuberculosis
2. Mycobacteria other than TB
3. SLE
4. Lung carcinoma
5. Bronchiectasis

THIS CXR SHOWS

Projection: PA, well centred, well penetrated, adequate field of view.

Irregular 3 cm LUZ opacity.

CLINICAL INTERPRETATION

Bronchoscopy revealed a tumour partially occluding the left upper lobe bronchus.

The subtle appearance of this lesion on the plain film, emphases the need to have a thorough and systematic method of reviewing chest x-rays in a busy clinical setting.

Systemic lupus erythematosus (SLE) has a number of pulmonary manifestations including pleural effusion, pleural pain and pulmonary fibrosis, but haemoptysis is exceedingly uncommon.

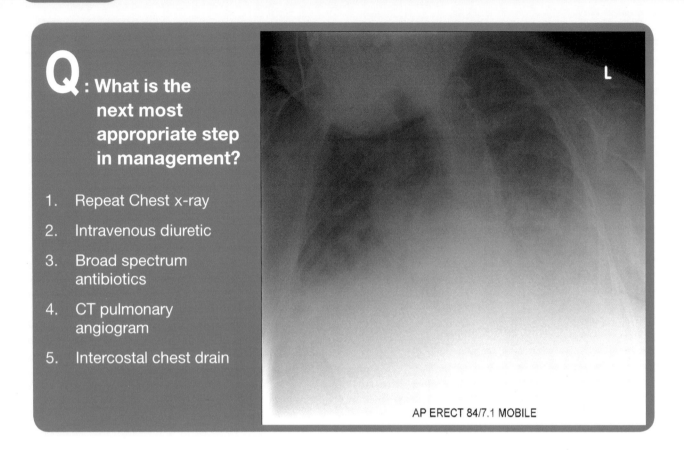

Q: What is the next most appropriate step in management?

1. Repeat Chest x-ray

2. Intravenous diuretic

3. Broad spectrum antibiotics

4. CT pulmonary angiogram

5. Intercostal chest drain

AP ERECT 84/7.1 MOBILE

THIS CXR SHOWS

Projection: AP, grossly rotated to the right, under penetrated, under inspired inadequate field of view

There is air space opacification bilaterally with lower zone predominance.

CLINICAL INTERPRETATION

WELCOME TO CLINICAL MEDICINE!

Poor films are unavoidable, particularly in sick in-patients and patients in a high dependency setting as most films are portable.

In addition, patients can be complex with multiple co-morbidities as in this lady's case. She suffered from rheumatoid arthritis, was treated with immunosuppressive therapy and had clinical evidence of decompensated cardiac failure. This made the differential diagnosis wide and challenging but intravenous diuretic is the most appropriate initial management.

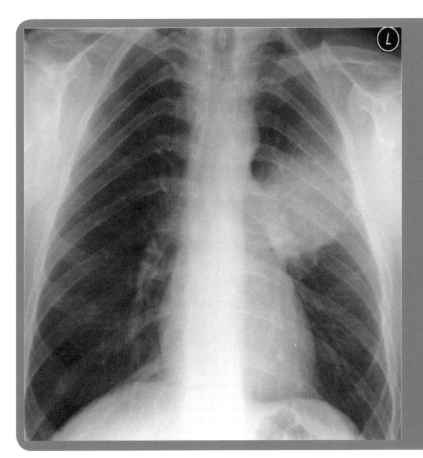

Q: Which feature is not evident on this chest x-ray?

1. Horizontal ribs

2. Left hilar mass

3. Increased bronchovascular markings

4. Hyperinflated lung fields

5. Pleural plaques

THIS CXR SHOWS

Projection: PA, well centred, adequate penetration. Apices and costophrenic angles not captured.

Hyperinflated lung fields with horizontal ribs but no flattening of the diaphragm. There is a large left hilar mass consistent with a bronchogenic carcinoma.

There are no pleural plaques.

CLINICAL INTERPRETATION

Bronchoscopy confirmed bronchogenic tumour, squamous cell type. Although the x-ray shows no pleural plaques or other evidence of asbestos disease, the patient was a carpenter with heavy previous exposure. He also smoked 30 cigarettes per day. The effects of asbestos exposure and cigarette smoke are additive - greatly increasing the individual's risk of lung cancer.[1]

[1] Doll R, Peto J. Asbestos: effects on health of exposure to asbestos. London: Health and Safety Commission, Her Majesty's Stationery Office, 1985:1-58

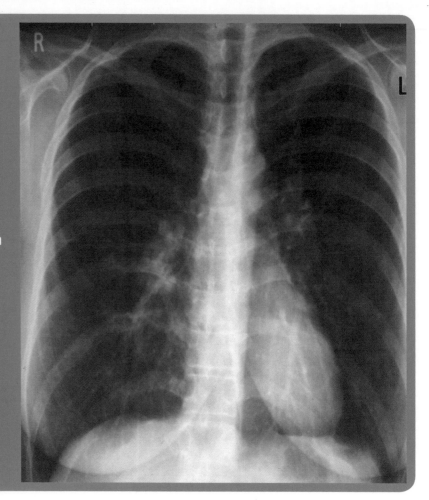

Q: What investigation is **unlikely** to help make the underlying diagnosis?

1. High resolution CT scan of chest

2. Static lung volumes

3. Transfer co-efficient

4. Serum ACE

5. Spirometry

THIS CXR SHOWS

Projection: PA, well centred, well penetrated, adequate field of view.

The lung fields are hyperinflated. There is paucity of lung markers in the upper zones consistent with emphysema. The pulmonary vasculature is prominent consistent with a degree of pulmonary hypertension.

CLINICAL INTERPRETATION

Hyperinflation is recognised by

- Greater than 7 anterior ribs or 10 posterior ribs visible above the diaphragm
- Relative flattening of the diaphragms
- The heart appears small, due to the increase in lung volume

Emphysema is characterised by dilation and destruction of the air-spaces distal to the terminal bronchioles; this destruction is recognised on chest x-ray by loss of the normal lung markings.

Patients may have obstructive spirometry, increased static lung volumes (particularly residual volume) and reduced transfer co-efficient.

Echocardiogram may show pulmonary hypertension.

Answer: 4) Serum ACE

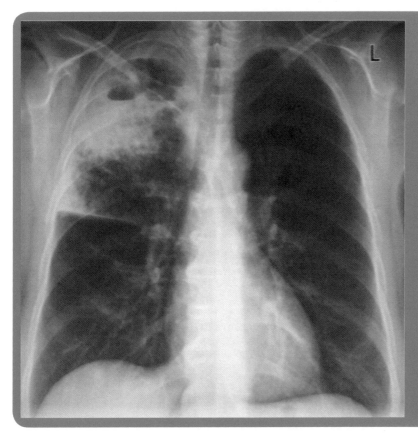

Q: Which of the following could **not** be responsible for this appearance?

1. Mycobacterium Tuberculosis

2. Squamous lung carcinoma

3. *Mycobacterium Kansasii*

4. *Klebsiella Pneumoniae*

5. Allergic bronchopulmonary aspergillosis (ABPA)

THIS CXR SHOWS

Projection: PA, well centred, well penetrated, adequate field of view.

There is widespread consolidation within the RUL demarcated by the horizontal fissure. There are multiple air-fluid levels consistent with cavities or multiple pulmonary abscesses.

CLINICAL INTERPRETATION

The differential diagnosis for pulmonary cavities or abscesses includes tuberculosis, staphylococcal and klebsiella pneumonia and squamous cell carcinoma.

Bronchial washings obtained at bronchoscopy showed squamous cell carcinoma as the cause of his cavitating disease.

Allergic bronchopulmonary aspergillosis does not cause cavitating disease. *Aspergillus fumigatus* can colonise pre-existing cavities causing an aspergilloma or chronic cavitatory aspergillosis.

Q: Which of the following would be appropriate treatment?

1. Intravenous beta-lactam and macrolide

2. Oral quinolone

3. IV heparin and CT pulmonary angiogram

4. Rifampicin and Clarithromycin

5. Intravenous ribavirin

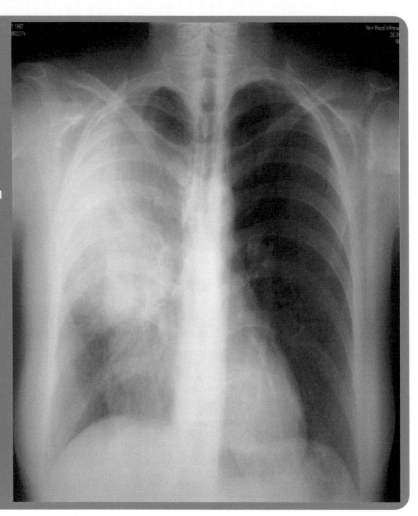

THIS CXR SHOWS

Projection: PA, well centred, well penetrated, adequate field of view.

Diffuse opacification throughout the right hemithorax with some sparing of the right lower zone.

The left lung is normal

CLINICAL INTERPRETATION

This previously healthy man presented with a severe community acquired pneumonia. The consolidation is not limited to a single anatomical lobe.

Multilobar pneumonia is associated with poor outcome.

Appropriate initial therapy for severe pneumonia is intravenous beta-lactam plus macrolide. Coverage of atypical organisms is associated with improved outcomes in severe pneumonia.[1]

[1] Am J Respir Crit Care Med. 2007 15;175(10):1086-93.

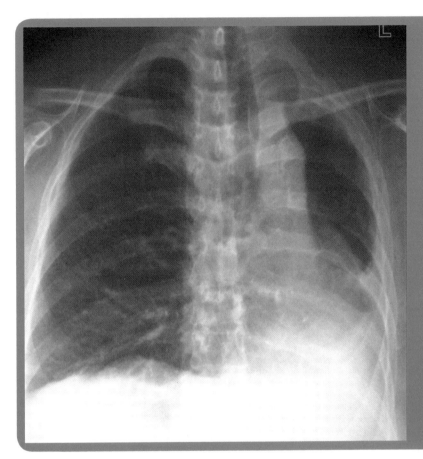

Q: What is the most likely cause of this CXR appearance?

1. Left pleural effusion

2. Left upper lobectomy

3. Left pneumonectomy

4. Right tension pneumothorax

5. Left lower lobe pneumonia

THIS CXR SHOWS

Projection: PA, well centred, over penetrated, adequate field of view.

The trachea and mediastinum are deviated to the left indicating a loss of volume in the left hemithorax. The changes are consistent with a left pneumonectomy. Bronchial wall thickening and dilatation consistent with bronchiectasis in the right lung

CLINICAL INTERPRETATION

This lady underwent a left pneumonectomy for localised bronchiectasis in the left lung. Unfortunately, she has also developed bronchiectasis in the right lung. Bronchiectasis is associated with a history of childhood respiratory infections, whooping cough and measles although the precise cause in most cases is not well understood.[1] Lobectomy and pneumonectomy may be indicated for severe localised bronchiectasis. Bronchiectasis is not easy to appreciate on a plain chest x-ray and is widely regarded as an HRCT diagnosis.

[1] Am J Respir Crit Care Med. 2000; 162(4 Pt 1):1277-84

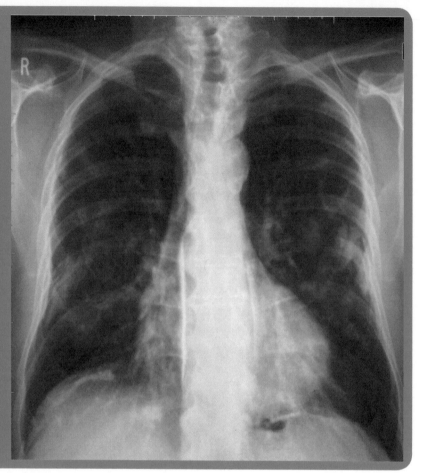

Q : Which of the following disorders is this patient not at increased risk of developing?

1. Pleural effusions

2. Mesothelioma

3. Bronchial carcinoma

4. Community acquired pneumonia

5. Pulmonary fibrosis

THIS CXR SHOWS

Projection: PA, some rotation to the right, well penetrated, adequate field of view.

There are calcified pleural plaques at both hemidiaphragms and in the mediastinum. The impression of opacification in both midzones is created by calcified pleural plaques sitting anteriorly on the pleural surface.

CLINICAL INTERPRETATION

Asbestos exposure causes 7 types of disease in the human lung

1. Asbestos bodies – recognised only at post-mortem and not seen on CXR

2. Pleural plaques - as shown

3. Asbestos related pleural thickening

4. Asbestos pleuritis- leading to recurrent pleural effusions

5. Asbestosis - pulmonary fibrosis (formally assessed on HRCT)

6. Malignant mesothelioma

7. Bronchial carcinoma

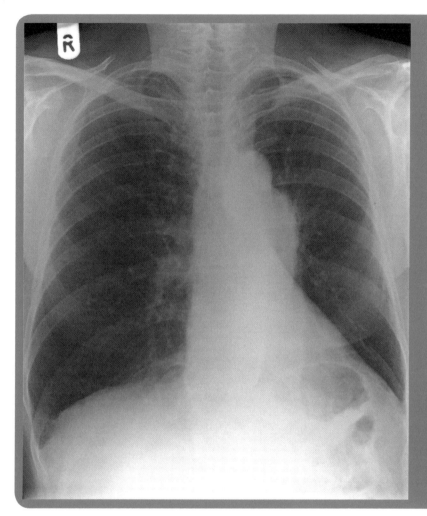

Q: What is the name given to this radiological sign?

1. The sail sign
2. Hamptons hump
3. De Mussets sign
4. Goldens "S" sign
5. Westermarks sign

THIS CXR SHOWS

Projection: PA, well centred, well penetrated, adequate field of view.

Superimposed breast shadows particularly on the left consistent with gynaecomastia. Left hilar mass with loss of volume on the left, triangular shaped dense opacity with obliteration of the left hemidiaphragm in keeping with left lower lobe collapse.

CLINICAL INTERPRETATION

This man has also lost weight and is a life long smoker. He has left lower lobe collapse on examination along with gynaecomastia which can be associated with lung and other malignancies. Bronchoscopy confirmed tumour obstructing the left lower lobe bronchus.

Retrocardiac opacities can easily be missed: careful examination of the retrocardiac space should always be a routine part of the chest film examination.

Q: Which of the following treatments would be inappropriate?

1. Surgical resection
2. Anti-fungal therapy
3. Bronchial artery embolisation
4. Tranexamic acid
5. Radical radiotherapy

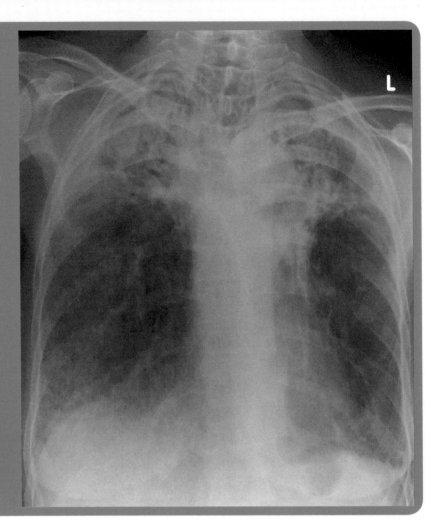

THIS CXR SHOWS

Projection: PA, well centred, well penetrated, adequate field of view.

Widespread interstitial opacification, predominantly at the bases with marked scarring and loss of volume in the upper zones.

There is a right apical cavity with a ball within.

CLINICAL INTERPRETATION

This lady has longstanding fibrotic lung disease, allergic bronchopulmonary aspergillosis and now has developed an aspergilloma in the right upper lobe (ball of fungal hyphae within a cavity in the lung).

Recurrent haemoptysis is common in patients with aspergilloma. Antifungal agents, treating bacterial infections and tranexamic acid may help. In some cases, arterial embolization or surgical resection may be required.

There is no evidence for the use of radiotherapy in this case.

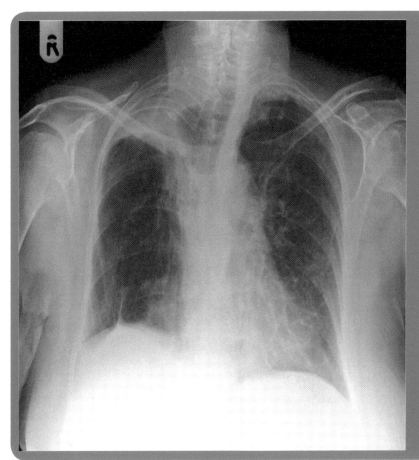

Q : The most likely cause of this appearance is:

1. *Mycobacterium Avium complex*

2. Right upper lobectomy

3. Bone metastasis from breast carcinoma

4. Aspergilloma

5. Silicosis

THIS CXR SHOWS

Projection: PA, well centred, well penetrated, adequate field of view.

There is loss of volume at the right apex with deviation of the trachea. The fifth rib has been resected suggesting a surgical right upper lobectomy. There are calcified foci in the left upper zone suggestive of old TB. There is scarring of the right lung base with compensatory emphysema.

CLINICAL INTERPRETATION

Evidence of old tuberculosis (TB) is relatively common in elderly patients presenting to medical assessment units. Surgical procedures used in the pre-antibiotic era included lobectomy (as in this case), thoracoplasty, plombage, phrenic nerve crush and pneumonectomy. The creation of artificial pneumothoraces were also used.

Old calcified granulomas are a common finding, however reactivation must be considered in the context of acute illness.

Q : Which of the following is the most likely diagnosis?

1. Right upper lobectomy

2. Hypersensitivity pneumonitis

3. Ankylosing spondylitis with upper zone fibrosis

4. Sarcoidosis

5. Cystic fibrosis

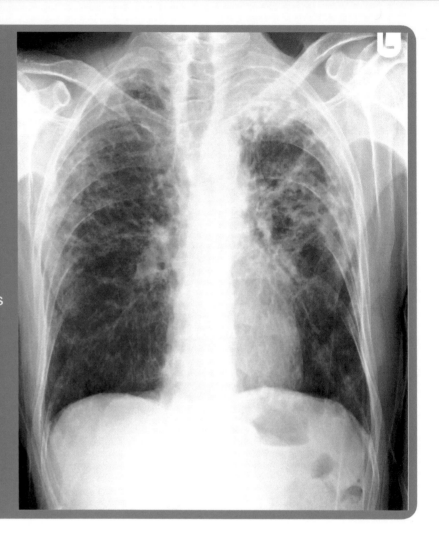

THIS CXR SHOWS

Projection: PA, well centred, well penetrated, adequate field of view.

There is widespread opacification throughout both lung fields greatest in the upper zones. The most striking abnormality is in the LUZ where there is homogenous opacification without obvious loss of volume. There is the impression of possible cavitation. There is pleural thickening. There are dilated bronchi visible suggestive of underlying bronchiectasis.

CLINICAL INTERPRETATION

This gentleman worked on a farm throughout his working life and describes episodes of acute breathlessness in the evenings following work, which resolved the following day. He has subsequently suffered with breathlessness and chronic sputum production throughout his adult life. The history is suggestive of extrinsic allergic alveolitis (Farmer's lung) which, when chronic, can lead to upper zone fibrosis. He has secondary bronchiectasis with chronic respiratory infections as a result.

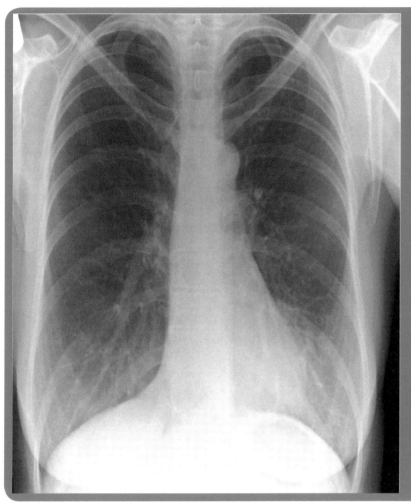

Q: Which pulmonary lobe does the lingula belong to?

1. RUL
2. RML
3. RLL
4. LUL
5. LLL

THIS CXR SHOWS

Projection: PA, well centred, well penetrated, adequate field of view.

Soft Tissues: Normal

Bones: Normal

Cardiac Silhouette: Loss of definition of the left heart border

Costophrenic Angles: Normal

Pulmonary: Normal

CLINICAL INTERPRETATION

Lingular consolidation is often missed; this x-ray appearance is frequently described as normal.

Loss of definition of the heart border signifies consolidation in the adjacent pulmonary tissue, in this case the lingula. Make sure your routine CXR examination includes a careful examination of heart, and diaphragmatic borders.

Q: What is the most appropriate next investigation?

1. Staging CT Thorax
2. Bronchoscopy
3. Sputum Culture
4. Pulmonary Function Tests
5. Gastroscopy

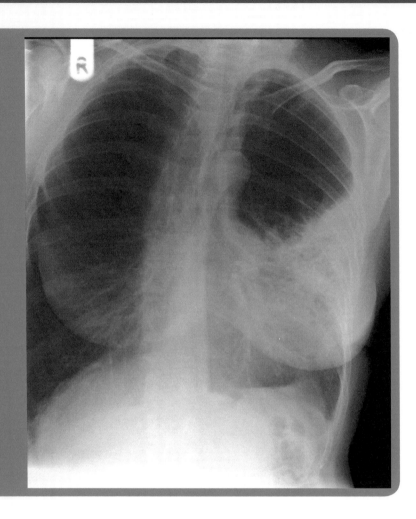

THIS CXR SHOWS

Projection: PA, adequate penetration, adequate field of view. There is marked kyphosis, convex to the right.

There is marked bullous emphysema with a large single bulla in the left upper zone.

There is significant airspace opacification in the left midzone, extending to the pleural surface, with adjacent volume loss.

CLINICAL INTERPRETATION

Airspace opacification is due to fluid within the alveolar spaces. This is most commonly secondary to infection, or pulmonary oedema. Unilateral airspace opacification is more likely to represent infection.

This lady had no symptoms of infection, raising the possibility of alternative aetiology. Staging CT of the thorax revealed a tumour at the origin of the left lower lobe bronchus.

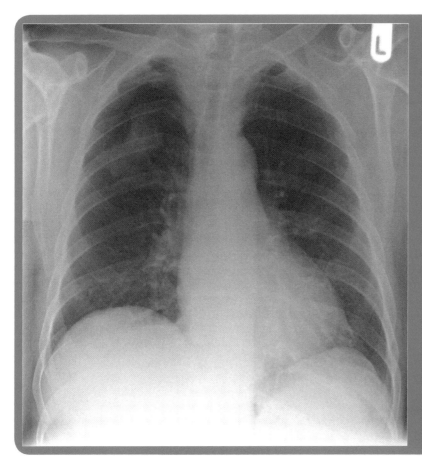

Q: What was the indication for the CT guided lung biopsy

1. Pleural effusion
2. Bronchial carcinoma
3. Hamartoma
4. Lung abscess
5. Cutaneous metastasis

THIS CXR SHOWS

Projection: PA, well centred, well penetrated, adequate field of view.

2.5 cm RUZ pneumothorax. Irregular RUL mass consistent with a bronchial carcinoma.

CLINICAL INTERPRETATION

CT guided lung biopsy is a mainstay investigation for sampling peripheral lung nodules.

There is high rate of pneumothorax, however only 10 % of such patients will require aspiration or intercostal drain insertion.[1]

Other complications include pulmonary haemorrhage, intercostal artery puncture, intercostal nerve damage.

Risk of death is estimated at 1:1000 and occurs due to introduction of air embolus into the pulmonary venous system.[1]

[1] Guidelines for radiologically guided lung biopsy
Thorax 2003; 58(11): 920 - 936

Q: What is the most **likely** pathogen?

1. Mycobacterium tuberculosis

2. Panton-Valentine Leucocidin positive *staphylococcus aureus*

3. Coagulase negative *staphylococcus aureus*

4. Pneumocystic Jirovecii

5. *Haemophilus influenzae*

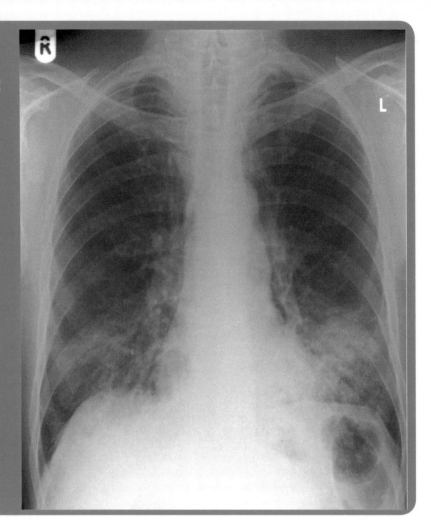

THIS CXR SHOWS

Projection: PA, well centred, under penetrated, adequate field of view.

There is bilateral airspace opacification in the lower zones, worse on the left.

CLINICAL INTERPRETATION

Airspace opacification in an immunosuppressed individual most likely represents pneumonia, and opportunistic infection must be considered. This man underwent bronchoscopy and bronchoalveolar lavage which confirmed the presence of *Pneumocystis Jirovecii*.

Treatment of Pneumocystis pneumonia is with high dose intravenous co-trimoxazole.

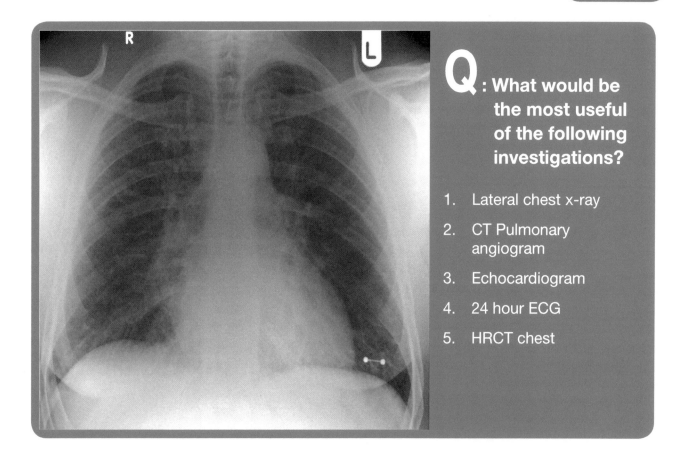

Q: What would be the most useful of the following investigations?

1. Lateral chest x-ray
2. CT Pulmonary angiogram
3. Echocardiogram
4. 24 hour ECG
5. HRCT chest

THIS CXR SHOWS

Projection: PA, well centred, well penetrated, adequate field of view.

Cardiac Silhouette: The cardiothoracic ratio is 180/160

There is a nipple bar through the left nipple

CLINICAL INTERPRETATION

There is significant cardiomegaly. In a previously fit young man the suspicion is of cardiomyopathy.

Echocardiography excluded hypertrophic obstructive cardiomyopathy, and confirmed a grossly dilated left ventricle.

This man has a history of anabolic steroid abuse, a rare cause of dilated cardiomyopathy.

Q: Which of the following would suggest empyema

1. C-reactive protein 91mg/l

2. Temperature 38.1°C

3. Pleural fluid LDH 770iu/L

4. Pleural fluid pH 7.12

5. Pleural fluid protein 50g/L

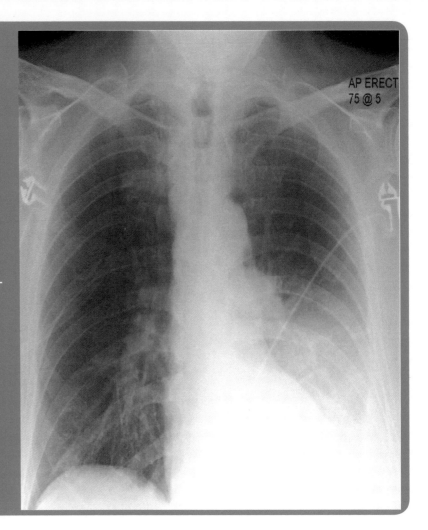

AP ERECT
75 @ 5

THIS CXR SHOWS

Projection: Portable AP film, well centred, under penetrated, adequate field of view.

The left hilum is prominent.

There is increased opacification at the left base with loss of the left diaphragmatic border.

There are ECG leads attached to the patient, and an oxygen mask and tubing are visible

CLINICAL INTERPRETATION

The changes represent a left sided pleural effusion. Pleural effusions are a common complication of pneumonia. Pleural aspiration revealed blood stained fluid, with a pH of 7.12. Intercostal tube drainage was carried out with good effect. Complicated parapneumonic effusions (those requiring urgent chest drainage) are defined by pH < 7.2, glucose < 2.2 mg / l or LDH > 1000 iu / ml.

The prominent left hilum was proven to be vascular prominence on CT imaging.

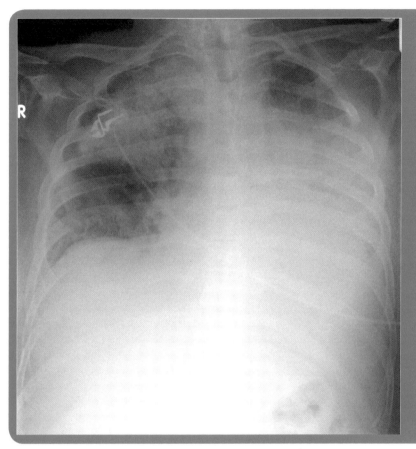

Q: Which of the following organisms is the most likely Cause of this appearance?

1. Methicillin resistant *staphylococcus aureus*

2. *Streptococcus Pneumoniae*

3. *Mycoplasma Pneumoniae*

4. *Moraxella Catarrhalis*

5. *Legionella Pneumophilia*

THIS CXR SHOWS

Projection: Portable AP film, slightly rotated to the right, under penetrated, and under inspired limiting field of view

There is increased opacification in the left base and midzone, with tracheal deviation to the left. There is airspace opacification in the RUZ, with air bronchograms visible.

CLINICAL INTERPRETATION

The film shows left sided volume loss, with consolidation in the right upper lobe.

Hospital Acquired Pneumonia may complicate a prolonged hospital stay. Lobar collapse may occur when a mucus plug obstructs a major airway. In contrast to community acquired pneumonia, multi-drug resistant pathogens (such as MRSA) and gram negative organisms predominate in hospital acquired pneumonia.[1] The prognosis is often poor, due to the organisms involved and the co-morbidities of the patients.

[1] Hospital-acquired pneumonia: risk factors, microbiology, and treatment. Chest. 2001;119(2 Suppl):373S-384S

Q: What is the most appropriate next investigation?

1. CT Thorax

2. Bronchoscopy

3. Pulmonary Function Tests

4. CT Abdomen

5. Urinalysis

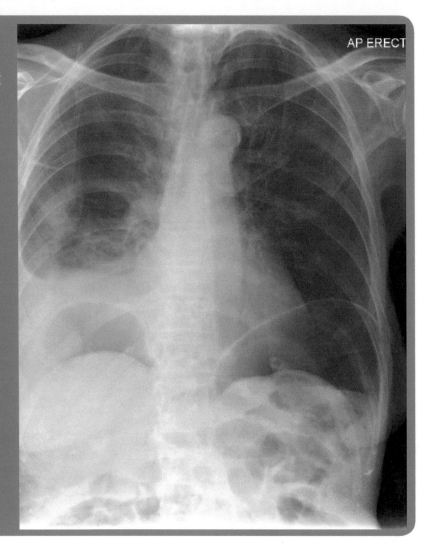

AP ERECT

THIS CXR SHOWS

Projection: PA, well centred, well penetrated, adequate field of view.

The film shows right lower lobe consolidation and a right sided pleural effusion. There is a large pneumoperitoneum.

CLINICAL INTERPRETATION

The right sided consolidation and effusion are due to infection, but do not explain her bilateral pain.

The presence of air beneath the diaphragm is pathological, unless the patient has recently undergone a laparoscopic procedure. In this case the pneumoperitoneum was due to a perforated diverticulum of the large bowel, and associated with bacterial peritonitis.

Dual contrast CT abdomen allows accurate localisation of the abnormality.

Answer: 4) CT Abdomen

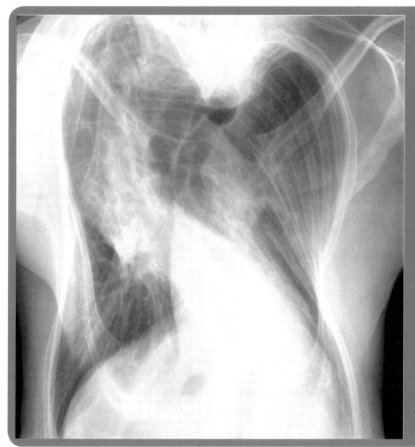

Q: What treatment might help this patients headache?

1. Paracetamol
2. Oral morphine solution
3. Continuous positive airway pressure (CPAP)
4. Bi-level Non-invasive ventilation
5. Lumbar punctures

THIS CXR SHOWS

Projection: PA, well centred, well penetrated, adequate field of view.

Severe kyphoscoliosis of the thoracic spine concave to the left in the upper portion of the thoracic cavity. As a result there is deformity of the ribs.

CLINICAL INTERPRETATION

This is a case of severe chest wall deformity. This leads to marked restriction of the patients dynamic lung volumes ultimately leading to alveolar hypoventilation and type 2 respiratory failure. This patient had high pCO_2 on morning arterial blood gas sampling. CO_2 retention causes headaches – the presence of hypercapnia and nocturnal hypoxaemia is an indication for non-invasive bi-level ventilation.

Q: Which pulmonary segment is affected?

1. Anterior segment RUL

2. Posterior segment RUL

3. Superior segment RML

4. Anterior segment RLL

5. Apical segment RLL

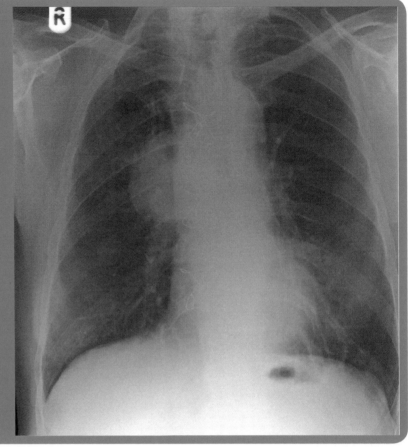

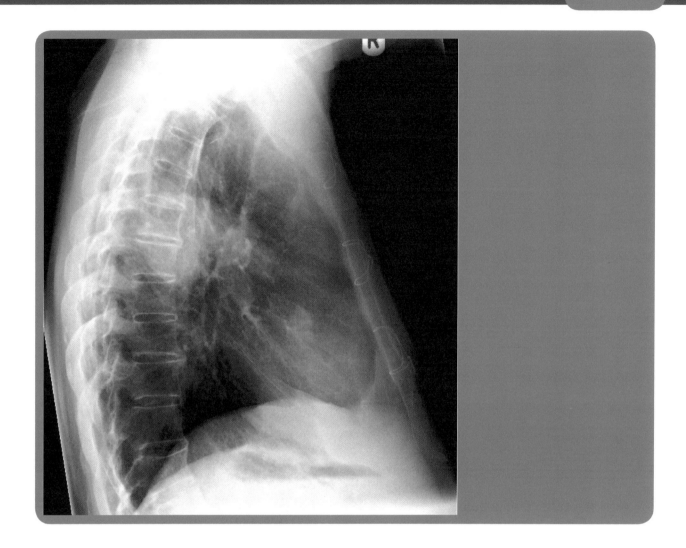

THIS CXR SHOWS

Projection: PA, centred, well penetrated, adequate field of view.

Sternotomy sutures present. 7 cm mass posterior to the right hilum (see right lateral film – apical segment of right lower lobe).

CLINICAL INTERPRETATION

Haemoptysis in a current, or ex, smoker is bronchogenic carcinoma until proven otherwise. Bronchoscopic evaluation is indicated here to confirm the diagnosis and the lateral film helps locate the tumour for targeted sampling in the unlikely event that no endobronchial lesion is visible. Staging CT chest provides a radiological staging, and guides further management.

Q: Which of the following CXR features commonly occurs in patients with alcohol mis-use?

1. Bilateral rib fractures

2. Widening of the mediastinum

3. Hiatus Hernia

4. Right lower lobe bronchiectasis

5. Bronchial carcinoma

THIS CXR SHOWS

Projection: PA, well centred, well penetrated, adequate field of view.

There is loss of volume of the right lung with collapse and likely pleural effusion.

Left lung clear.

CLINICAL INTERPRETATION

CT scanning of the thorax confirmed RLL collapse, pleural effusion, but did not demonstrate endobronchial lesion. Bronchoscopy was also normal. Clinically, he was an unkempt individual, had a history of heavy alcohol consumption along with clinical stigmata of chronic liver disease, ascites and a transudate pleural effusion in keeping with a diagnosis of hepatic hydrothorax.

He was relieved that no "cancer" was found and was planning to go out for a drink to celebrate!

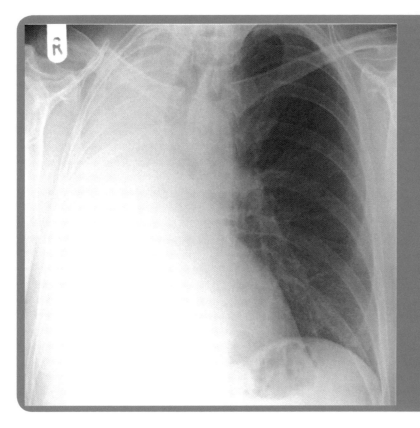

Q: Which of the following diagnoses could explain this appearance?

1. Pulmonary embolism

2. RLL Lobectomy

3. Right main bronchus carcinoma

4. Mucous plugging RLL

5. Aspiration pneumonia

THIS CXR SHOWS

Projection: PA, well centred, well penetrated, adequate field of view.

Complete white out of the right lung field with shifting of the mediastinum towards the right.

Clear left lung field.

CLINICAL INTERPRETATION

There are 3 main causes of complete "white out" on the CXR: pneumonectomy; total lung collapse; and pleural effusion. In the latter, the mediastinum is shifted away from the pathological lung. Compare this chest x-ray with Case 2 to see how to differentiate collapse and effusion in a "white-out".

This CXR shows a right lung collapse and in a patient with progressive breathlessness this suggests a proximal obstructing lesion.

Q: How would you describe the abnormality on this chest film?

1. Micro-nodular opacification
2. Reticular-nodular shadowing
3. Air-bronchograms
4. Upper lobe venous diversion
5. Bilateral hilar lymphadenopathy

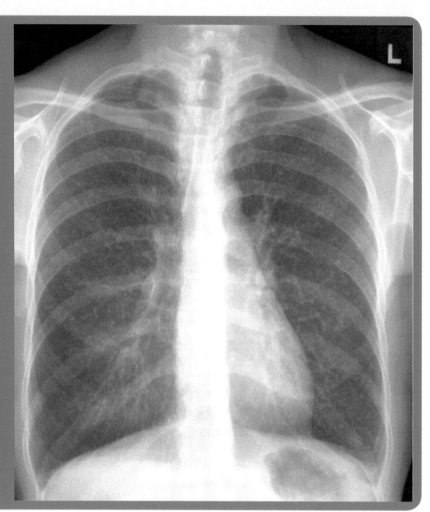

THIS CXR SHOWS

Projection: PA, well centred, well penetrated, adequate field of view.

Small calcified nodules scattered throughout both lung fields.

CLINICAL INTERPRETATION

This lady has had previous chicken pox pneumonitis and has been left with these small calcified nodules. This should not impinge on her respiratory reserve and her asthma should be managed conventionally. The junior doctor had requested a CXR to rule out a pneumothorax and was concerned about the findings of this CXR. She and the patient were quickly reassured!

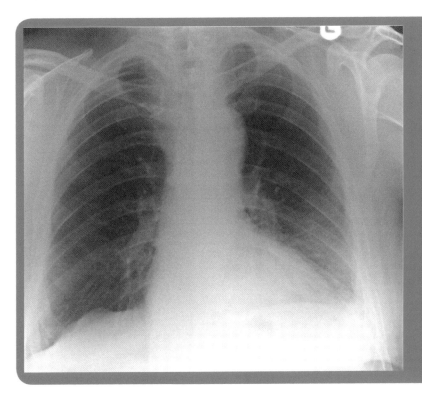

Q : What is the diagnosis?

1. Right mid zone bronchial carcinoma

2. Community Acquired Pneumonia

3. Right lung abscess

4. Normal chest x-ray other than eventration of the right hemi-diaphragm

5. Right upper lobe collapse due to TB

THIS CXR SHOWS

Projection: PA, slight rotation to the left, well penetrated, adequate field of view.

RMZ 1 cm well defined opacity with a hypolucent centre consistent with a button.

The left hemidiaphragm is elevated with patchy opacification consistent with a left lower lobe pneumonia.

CLINICAL INTERPRETATION

The patient presented with a left lower lobe pneumonia. In an ex-smoker it was quite reasonable for the house officer to question whether there might be an associated mass. Remember, the x-ray doesn't just image the lungs. Prior to seeing the respiratory team this patient already had a CT chest performed which confirmed a left lower lobe pneumonia with no other abnormalities.

Q: Which of the following would be appropriate treatment in this case?

1. Chest physiotherapy
2. Intravenous broad-spectrum antibiotics
3. Nebulised antibiotics
4. Pulmonary rehabilitation
5. All of the above

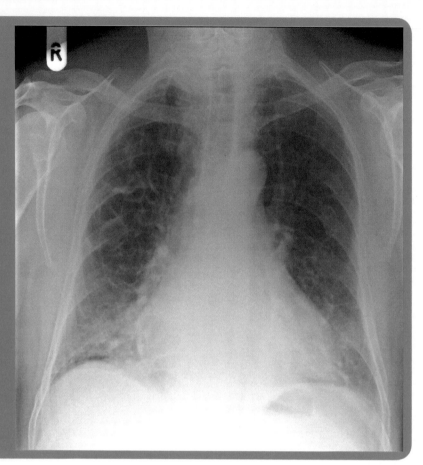

THIS CXR SHOWS

Projection: PA, well centred, slightly under penetrated, adequate field of view.

There are multiple thin walled cysts in the RUL some of which contain fluid. There is peribronchial thickening in the right and left lower lobes. There is slight cardiomegaly and incidental finding of old left sided rib fractures. The appearances are consistent with severe cystic bronchiectasis

CLINICAL INTERPRETATION

Bronchiectasis is permanent dilation of the bronchi and presents with recurrent chest infections and chronic production of (usually) purulent sputum. This man clearly has very severe bronchiectasis with cyst formation. Patients with severe bronchiectasis are often colonised with organisms such as *pseudomonas aeruginosa*. The mainstays of therapy are antibiotics for exacerbations, chest clearance techniques (physiotherapy) and sometimes nebulised antibiotics (as were used in this case).

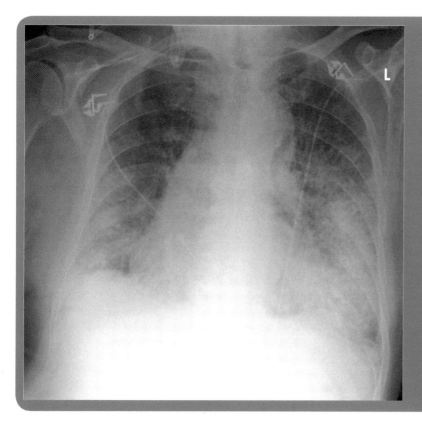

Q: Which of the following is the most likely ECG finding?

1. AV nodal re-entry tachycardia

2. Left bundle branch block

3. Right bundle branch block

4. S1 Q3 T3

5. Second degree heart block

THIS CXR SHOWS

Projection: Supine erect AP, rotated to the right, under penetrated, adequate field of view.

Bilateral airspace opacification MZ and LZ left more than right with Kerley B lines, blunting of the right costophrenic angle, cardiomegaly and upper lobe venous distension.

CLINICAL INTERPRETATION

Acute pulmonary oedema. This man, known to have ischaemic heart disease, was recently discharged from hospital following admission with decompensated heart failure. He responded well to nitrate infusion, iv morphine, iv diuretics and continuous positive airway pressure (CPAP) therapy. This episode of decompensation was secondary to ST elevation myocardial infarction, a common cause of acute pulmonary oedema.

Q: What is the most likely primary tumour?

1. Osteosarcoma
2. Pancreatic carcinoma
3. Angiosarcoma
4. Mesothelioma
5. Renal Cell Carcinoma

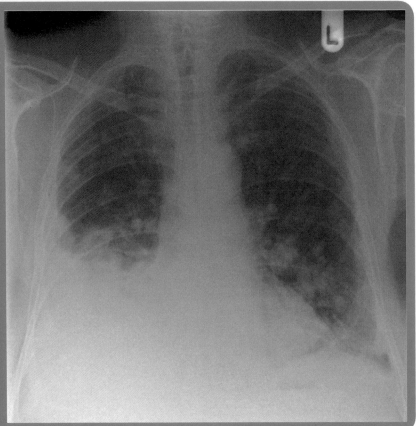

THIS CXR SHOWS

Projection: PA, well centred, well penetrated, adequate field of view.

Fracture left 8th posterior rib. Multiple "cannon ball" round soft tissue opacities throughout both lungs.

Right pleural effusion

CLINICAL INTERPRETATION

This man has progressive disseminated renal carcinoma with breathlessness secondary to pleural effusion and pulmonary metastases. Palliative intercostal drainage may help relieve this man's symptoms.

Renal cell carcinoma presents insidiously and is often diagnosed on the basis of this chest x-ray appearance, which is virtually pathognomonic.

Answer: 5) Renal cell carcinoma ★ ★

This 73 year old retired plumber underwent a CXR after presenting with right sided chest discomfort.

CXR 39

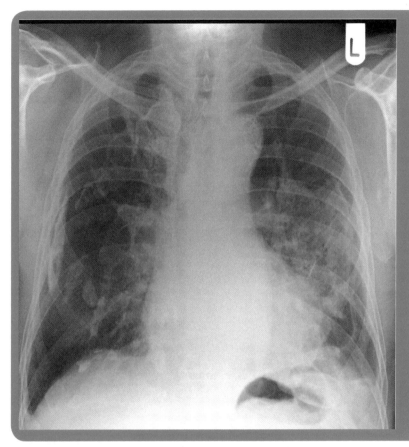

Q: Which of the following disorders is usually asymptomatic?

1. Asbestosis

2. Mesothelioma

3. Asbestosis related pleural thickening

4. Pleural Plaques

5. Asbestos related lung carcinoma

THIS CXR SHOWS

Projection: PA, well centred, well penetrated, adequate field of view.

There are widespread, large, irregular calcified pleural based opacities overlying the diaphragms and lung fields. There is also bilateral blunting of the costophrenic angles which suggests pleural effusions or long standing pleural thickening.

CLINICAL INTERPRETATION

The CXR findings of pleural plaques and pleural thickening are often made incidentally. Pleural plaques infrequently cause symptoms. In the United Kingdom, as of March 2009 one can claim compensation for pleural thickening and other asbestos related disease but not for asymptomatic pleural plaques alone. Pleural plaques can be considered to be a marker of significant asbestos exposure, but do not increase the risk of development of mesothelioma, per se.

Pleural plaques are usually asymptomatic.

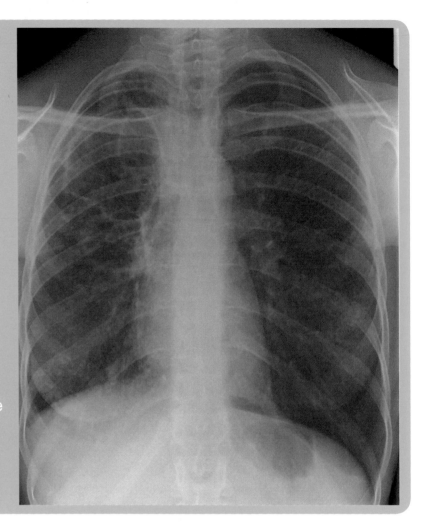

Q : What is the most appropriate next step?

1. Empirical anti-tuberculous chemotherapy

2. Low molecular weight heparin and urgent CT pulmonary angiogram

3. Intravenous ceftazidime and Gentamicin for 2 weeks

4. IV ribavirin

5. Send sputum for culture

THIS CXR SHOWS

Projection: PA, well centred, well penetrated, adequate field of view.

RUZ cavitation with diffuse miliary type shadowing throughout both lung fields.

CLINICAL INTERPRETATION

Mycobacerial Tuberculosis is the most likely diagnosis and empirical quadruple anti-tuberculous chemotherapy should be commenced. The diagnosis is confirmed by detection of acid and alcohol fast bacilli in sputum or bronchial washing samples, or positive culture of mycobacteria. Miliary (or disseminated) TB is thankfully rare, accounting for 1-2% of TB cases. Lesions are spread throughout the body, particularly in the lungs, liver and spleen. The name arises from the chest x-ray appearance which has been likened to millet seeds.

65 year old man who was treated for bronchoalveolar carcinoma presents with cough secondary to rape seed oil allergy.

CXR 41

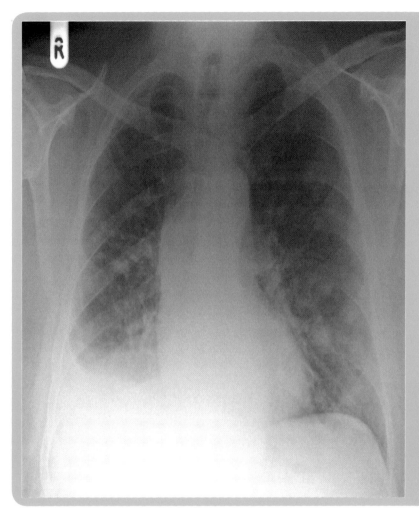

Q: Which of the following features are not present on this chest x-ray?

1. Pleural effusion
2. Right hilar enlargement
3. Multiple rounded opacities
4. Under-penetration
5. Left atrial enlargement

THIS CXR SHOWS

Projection: PA, well centred, under penetrated, adequate field of view.

Right Hilar enlargement

Right pleural effusion. Multiple, widespread round soft tissue opacities suggestive of pleural metastasis.

CLINICAL INTERPRETATION

Bronchoalveolar carcinoma is a particularly aggressive type of carcinoma and is fortunately rare making up < 1% of all lung cancers. Most patients have tumour spread at presentation.

Detection of bronchoalveolar carcinoma is difficult: CT scan appearances may mimic infection; bronchoscopic appearances are often normal; pathological confirmation requires transbronchial biopsy.

Q : This x-ray shows:

1. Diaphragmatic hernia
2. Left pleural effusion
3. Left ventricular enlargement
4. Left atrial enlargement
5. Cystic splenic mass

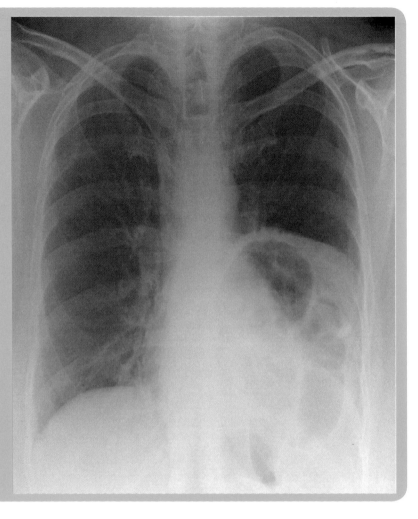

THIS CXR SHOWS

Projection: PA, well centred, well penetrated, adequate field of view.

There is elevation of the left hemidiaphragm with a large incarcerated hiatus hernia. The lung fields are clear.

CLINICAL INTERPRETATION

The patient complained of severe heartburn. Her stomach appears to lie within the thoracic cavity; barium swallow and upper GI endoscopy confirmed the stomach to be above the diaphragm. Hiatus hernia is not an uncommon finding on a chest x-ray but is usually of no pathological significance. However, gastric reflux, frequently associated with hiatus hernia, is strongly associated with chronic cough.

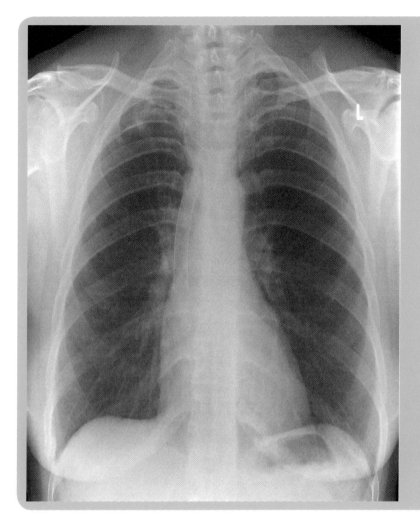

Q : What was her presenting complaint?

1. Chest pain
2. Haemoptysis
3. Fever and night sweats
4. Facial swelling
5. Erythema nodosum

THIS CXR SHOWS

Projection: PA, well centred, well penetrated, adequate field of view.

There is an opacity in the RUL overlying the rib. There is a superior vena cava stent in situ.

CLINICAL INTERPRETATION

This patient presented with facial swelling as a consequence of superior vena cava obstruction (SVCO). The diagnosis is small cell lung cancer. CT chest demonstrated a large mediastinal mass compressing the SVC. SVCO is recognised by facial swelling and the appearance of dilated veins over the upper chest and face. Treatment is usually with dexamethasone, stent insertion and palliative radiotherapy.

Q : Which of the following tests may make the diagnosis?

1. Echocardiogram
2. Sweat test
3. Urinary free cortisol
4. Semen analysis
5. Serum α-1 antitrypsin

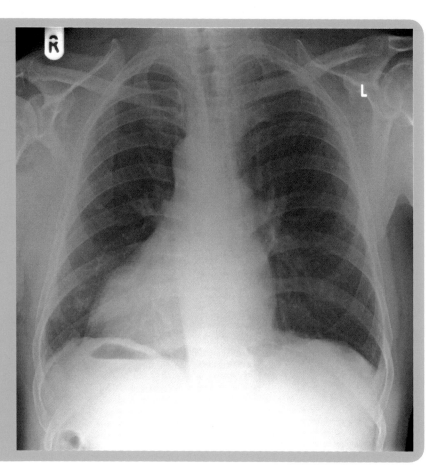

THIS CXR SHOWS

Projection: PA, right rotation, well penetrated, adequate field of view.

The lung fields are clear. There is *situs invertus.* The heart and aortic shadow are on the right and the appearance of the gastric bubble beneath the right hemidiaphragm confirms complete *situs invertus.*

CLINICAL INTERPRETATION

Situs invertus literally means that all of the organs are "the wrong way round". The heart and stomach are on the right side of the body and the left hemidiaphragm is higher than on the right indicating a left sided liver. *Situs invertus* is linked to a number of disorders, but in a patient with cough the likely diagnosis is Kartagener's syndrome - the combination of primary ciliary dyskinesia (manifesting as sinusitis and bronchiectasis) with *situs invertus.*

Patients have immotile sperm due to ciliary dysfunction.

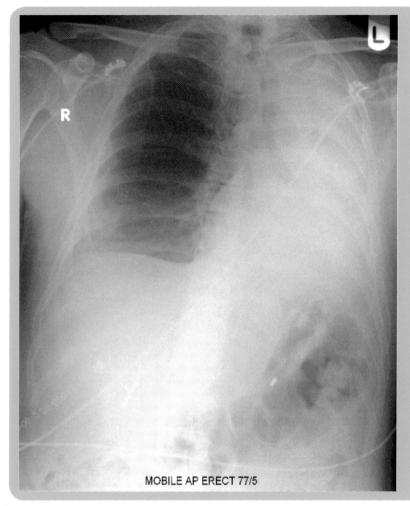

MOBILE AP ERECT 77/5

Q: What intervention may relieve this patients symptoms?

1. Intercostal chest drain

2. LMWH and CT pulmonary angiogram

3. Ryles tube

4. Bronchoscopy

5. Ureteric stent

THIS CXR SHOWS

Projection: AP, centred, over penetrated, adequate field of view.

There is complete white out of the left lung with mediastinal shift to the left suggestive of left lung collapse as the cause.

CLINICAL INTERPRETATION

Lobar collapse due to secretions is relatively common post-operatively: anaesthesia compromises natural mechanisms of airway clearance. At bronchoscopy the left main bronchus was occluded with viscous secretions – these secretions were suctioned during the procedure. Post procedure chest x-ray showed re-inflation of the lung, and the patient had symptomatic relief.

Q : The following investigations and treatment are useful in this disease **except:**

1. Bronchial artery embolisation

2. Urinalysis

3. Intravenous corticosteroids

4. Bronchoscopy

5. Thiopurine methyltransferase blood assay

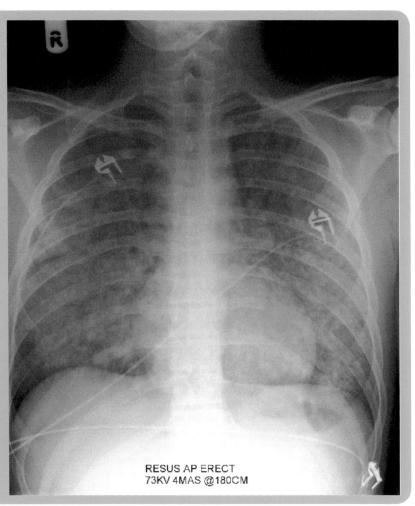

RESUS AP ERECT
73KV 4MAS @180CM

THIS CXR SHOWS

CLINICAL INTERPRETATION

Projection: AP, well centred, well penetrated, adequate field of view.

There is patchy air-space opacification throughout both lung fields and affecting all zones.

This young man presented with large volume haemoptysis and consequent severe anaemia. The chest x-ray appearances are typical of pulmonary haemorrhage and as expected, a large volume of blood was seen throughout the bronchial tree at bronchoscopy. The cause was systemic vasculitis. Disorders such as Goodpastures syndrome (anti-glomerular basement membrane disease) and Wegeners granulomatosis may present with pulmonary haemorrhage and are invariably associated with haematuria. Massive pulmonary haemorrhage is usually bronchial rather than alveolar in origin, however this was a severe case of the latter.

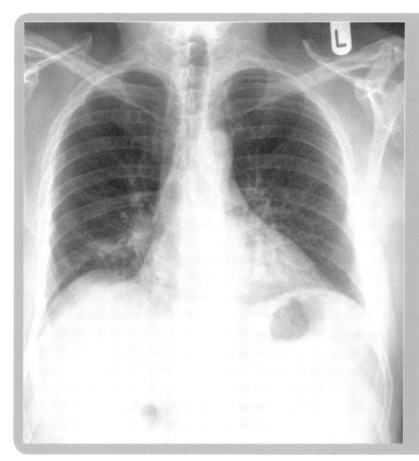

Q: Which of the following investigations is routinely used prior to surgery for staging of lung cancer?

1. Sputum cytology

2. Positron Emission Tomography (PET)

3. CT pulmonary angiogram

4. CT brain

5. Isotope bone scan

THIS CXR SHOWS

Projection: PA, well centred, adequately penetrated, under-inspired film.

There is loss of volume on the right associated with some opacification below the right hilum. The rest of the lungs are clear.

CLINICAL INTERPRETATION

This gentleman presented with jaundice 6 months after a middle lobectomy for early stage lung cancer. Before being considered for surgical treatment patients undergo full radiological staging with CT and PET scanning to exclude distant metastases. Unfortunately, these methods do not have a 100 % negative predictive value for excluding small metastases and this man's presentation raises the possibility of occult metastatic disease.

The combination of PET and CT for staging lung cancer is 93% sensitive and 97% specific.

[1] N Engl J Med. 2003; 19;348(25):2500-7

Q: The abnormality is in...?

1. The left lower lobe
2. The right upper lobe
3. The anterior mediastinum
4. Below the diaphragm
5. No-where, it's a normal appearance

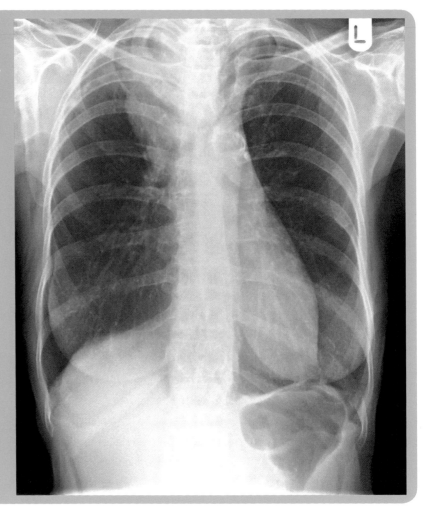

THIS CXR SHOWS

Projection: PA, well centred, well penetrated, adequate field of view.

There is a 7 cm mass in the superior mediastinum and medial part of the right upper zone. It displaces the trachea to the right

CLINICAL INTERPRETATION

The abnormality lies either in the superior mediastinum, or the right upper lobe, or both. In a smoker the most likely diagnosis is lung cancer, and given the volume loss in the right lung, on balance this is more likely to be a lung tumour with mediastinal invasion than a mediastinal primary malignancy.

At bronchoscopy the right upper lobe bronchus was obstructed at its origin, and biopsies confirmed non small-cell lung cancer.

In cases such as this, there is no substitute for a biopsy!

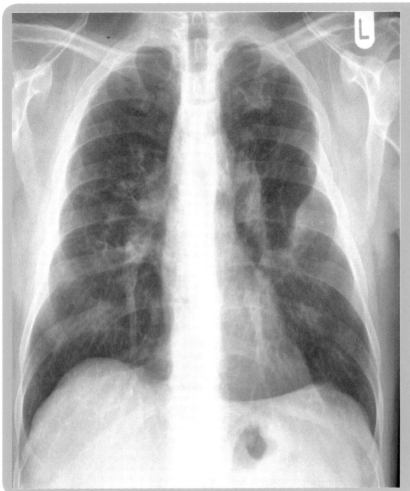

Q: Which of the following investigations would not be useful in this case?

1. Serum calcium

2. High resolution CT chest

3. Pulmonary artery catheterisation

4. Skin biopsy

5. Transbronchial lung biopsy

THIS CXR SHOWS

Projection: PA, well centred, well penetrated, adequate field of view.

There is striking bilateral hilar lymphadenopathy. There is also increased opacification in the mid and upper zones bilaterally consistent with interstitial change. There is some tethering of the left hemidiaphragm of no clinical significance.

CLINICAL INTERPRETATION

The appearances are classical of stage 2 sarcoidosis (bilateral hilar lymphadenopathy with interstitial changes). Compare with case 5.

Calcium may be elevated in sarcoidosis due to production of vitamin D by macrophages. HRCT chest will characterise the interstitial involvement. Skin biopsy may be helpful in erythema nodosum or lupus pernio. Transbronchial lung biopsy is often used to confirm sarcoidosis and may show typical non-caeseating granulomas.

Q : What other past medical history does this lady have?

1. Aspergilloma

2. Invasive aspergillosis

3. Right sided empyema

4. Pulmonary tuberculosis

5. Right upper lobectomy for lung carcinoma

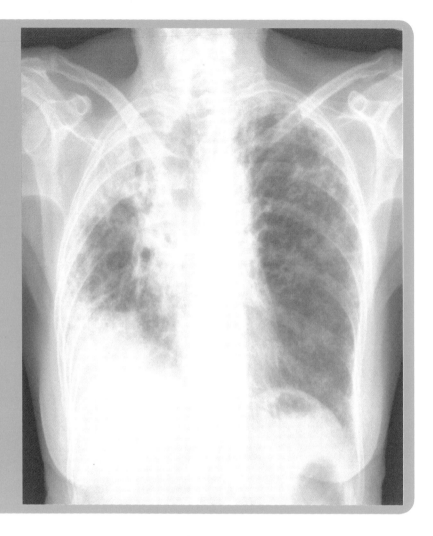

THIS CXR SHOWS

Projection: PA, well centred, under penetrated, adequate field of view.

The trachea is deviated to the right and there is loss of volume in the RUL. There is evidence of fibrosis and pleural thickening in the RUL. There is also LUZ opacity in keeping with a degree of fibrosis.

CLINICAL INTERPRETATION

The right sided appearances are typical of post radiation therapy fibrosis, in this case for lymphoma. The LUZ changes are due to previous tuberculosis. Without the history of lymphoma, you might have thought that these changes were entirely due to previous tuberculosis. As always, the history is everything.

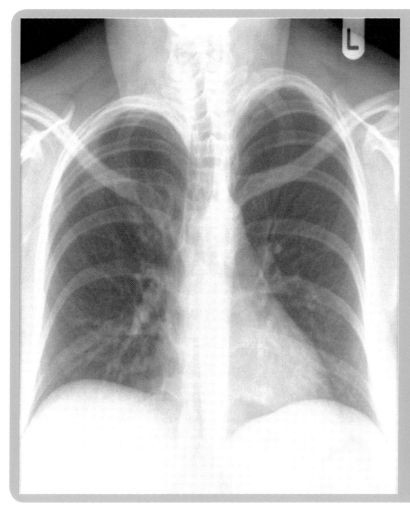

Q: Which of the following is not a risk factor for MRSA septicaemia?

1. Central venous catheter

2. Arterial line

3. Venous leg ulcer

4. COPD

5. Hospital acquired Pneumonia

THIS CXR SHOWS

Projection: PA, well penetrated, adequate field of view.

Kyphoscoliosis evident. There is an intravenous line arising from the right arm the tip of which most likely lies in the right atrium.

CLINICAL INTERPRETATION

This patient was receiving intravenous anti-arrythmic therapy via a peripherally inserted central venous catheter (PICC line). Long lines are an important cause of hospital acquired infection as in this case.

The ideal position for the tip of any central venous catheter is the junction of the SVC and the right atrium. At this point the high blood flow reduces the risk of clot formation at the line tip.

Q: The chest x-ray shows

1. Lung abscess
2. Empyema
3. Hydropneumothorax
4. Pleural thickening
5. Mesothelioma

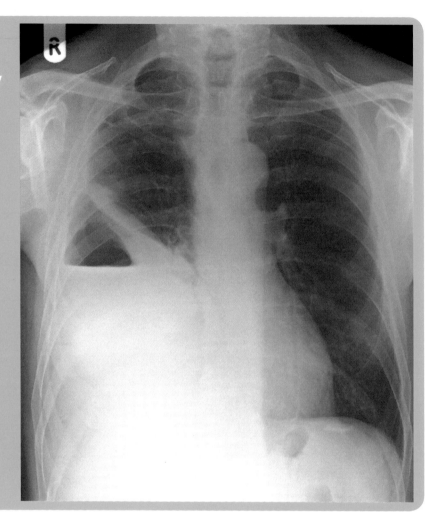

THIS CXR SHOWS

Projection: PA, well centred, under penetrated, adequate field of view.

There is a large right sided pleural effusion with an air fluid level clearly visible in the RMZ. This is consistent with a hydropneumothorax. There is some emphysema in the upper lobes but the rest of the lung fields are clear.

CLINICAL INTERPRETATION

The x-ray shows a hydropneumothorax.

The differential diagnosis for this appearance includes cavitating lung carcinoma, lung abscess and empyema. This gentleman had developed right sided chest pain on holiday in Spain and had not sought medical attention. Aspiration of the pleural space revealed foul-smelling, frank pus, which grew gram negative bacteria on culture. These gas forming organisms are responsible for the air visible on the admission chest-x-ray. He was treated with intravenous antibiotics and intercostal drainage, and made a full recovery.

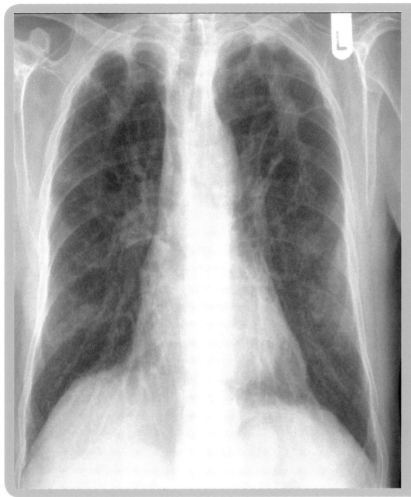

Q: What test may help determine the severity of this mans disease?

1. Diffusing capacity of carbon monoxide (DLCO)

2. Specific IgE to Aspergillus

3. Mycopolyspora Faeni IgG

4. Avian Precipitin Titre

5. Exhaled nitric oxide

THIS CXR SHOWS

Projection: PA, well centred, adequately penetrated, adequate field of view.

There is increased opacity in the upper and midzones bilaterally, with relative sparing of the bases. The opacities coalesce into more rounded soft tissue lesions in the upper zones.

CLINICAL INTERPRETATION

This gentleman has upper and mid zone fibrosis and an elevated serum IgG to pigeons consistent with the clinical diagnosis of bird fanciers lung. Extrinsic allergic alveolitis is a chronic hypersensitivity pneumonitis due to repeated exposure to an antigen, in this case bird allergen.

The differential diagnosis for upper zone fibrosis is: Sarcoidosis, extrinsic allergic alveolitis, ankylosing spondylitis and tuberculosis.

Q : The following can be associated with this disease **except:**

1. Epistaxis
2. Dysphagia
3. Seizures
4. Brain abscess
5. Jaundice

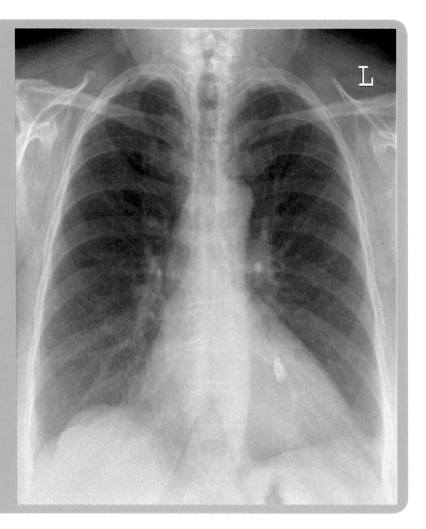

THIS CXR SHOWS

Projection: PA, well centred, well penetrated, adequate field of view.

There is generalised increase in lung markers but no active pulmonary lesion is identified. The most obvious finding is the radio-opaque density behind the heart border.

CLINICAL INTERPRETATION

Hereditary haemorrhagic telangiectasia (Osler Weber Rendu syndrome) is associated with pulmonary arteriovenous malformations (AVM) – as the vasculature is fragile, these can rupture, leading to recurrent haemoptysis as they did in this case. Treatment is by embolisation, or by resection for larger AVMs. The opacity behind the heart is an embolisation coil.

HHT is associated with recurrent epistaxis, neurological complications including seizure, brain abscesses and stroke. Liver involvement may be asymptomatic but can cause jaundice or abdominal pain.

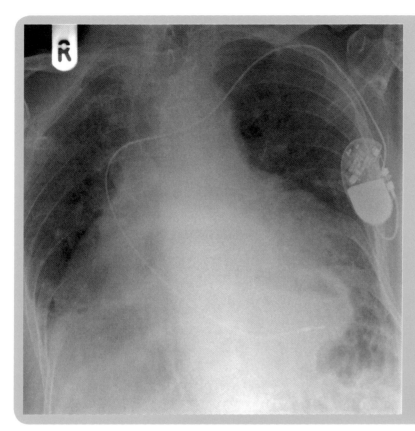

Q : Cardiomegaly on the chest x-ray can be due to all the following except:

1. Pericardial effusion
2. Left ventricular aneurysm
3. Dilated cardiomyopathy
4. Dissected thoracic aortic aneurysm
5. Mitral stenosis

THIS CXR SHOWS

Projection: PA, off centre, under penetrated, under inspired.

Gross cardiomegaly and single chamber pacemaker in situ

CLINICAL INTERPRETATION

This lady had a history of brady-arrhythmia treated with a permanent pacemaker. The pacemaker was functioning normally. Her breathlessness was due to left ventricular dysfunction which was optimised medically.

Dissecting thoracic aortic aneurysm can cause apparent cardiac enlargement due to haemopericardium. Mitral stenosis typically is not associated with left ventricular enlargement.

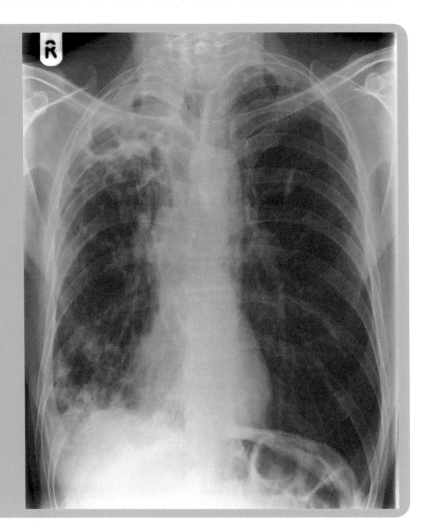

Q: Which of the following investigations would be most appropriate?

1. Interferon gamma assay

2. Heaf test

3. CT chest

4. Sputum Acid and Alcohol Fast Bacilli (AAFB)

5. Sputum cytology

THIS CXR SHOWS

Projection: PA, well centred, well penetrated, adequate field of view.

There is loss of volume of the RUL and deviation of the trachea to the right. There is fibrosis and cavitation in the RUL. There is also some inflammatory change at the right lung base. The left lung is clear.

CLINICAL INTERPRETATION

The history of weight loss in association with these x-ray appearances are highly suggestive of further mycobacterial disease. This gentleman had tuberculosis in his youth and a subsequent RUL cavity. Although reactivation of previous tuberculosis was suspected, the cavity had been secondarily infected by *Mycobacterium Malmoense*, an opportunistic mycobacteria. Opportunistic mycobacteria are ubiquitous organisms that usually only cause disease in patients with chronically damaged lungs. It is only possible to distinguish tuberculosis from other mycobacterial diseases by microbiological examination of infected sputum, bronchial washings, or histology. Opportunistic mycobacteria are invariably resistant to a variety of antibiotics, and prolonged treatment with multiple agents is required.

Answer: 4) Sputum Acid and Alcohol Fast Bacilli (AAFB)

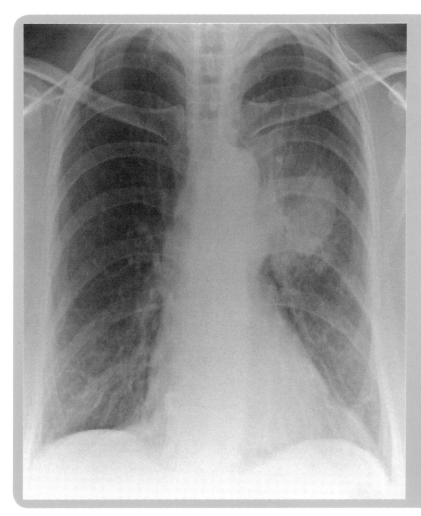

Q: What would best describe the location of this lesion?

1. LUL
2. Lingula
3. LLL
4. LMZ
5. LLZ

THIS CXR SHOWS

Projection: PA, well centred, adequately penetrated, apices not fully captured in field of view

Increased cardiothoracic ratio. There is a 6 cm mass extending from the left hilum with surrounding patchy opacification possibly due to surrounding consolidation.

CLINICAL INTERPRETATION

Given the central location of the abnormality, bronchoscopy was arranged, however no endobronchial lesion was seen. CT revealed an 8 x 8 cm mass within the apical segment of the left lower lobe. CT guided lung biopsy confirmed non-small cell lung cancer. Remember that the lower lobes extend through the midzones and into the upper zones on a chest X-Ray; without a lateral film, or a CT, it is often difficult to give an accurate anatomical location – when describing a CXR stick to zones!

Q: Which of the following is not a common site for lung cancer metastases?

1. Adrenal gland
2. Bone
3. Liver
4. Lung
5. Kidney

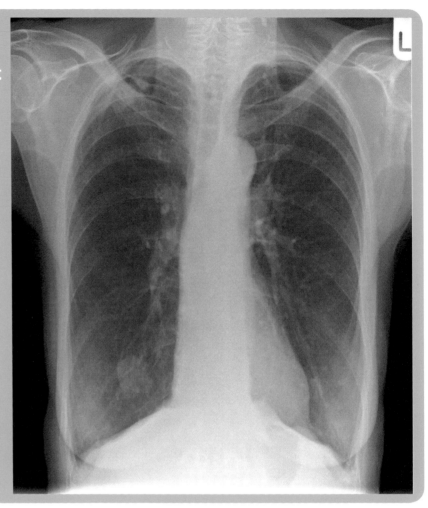

THIS CXR SHOWS

Projection: PA, well centred, adequate penetration, adequate field of view.

There are background changes consistent with COPD. There are bilateral upper zone changes with a calcified left cervical node suggestive of old TB. There is a 3cm round mass in the RLZ.

CLINICAL INTERPRETATION

The appearances are of a right lower zone bronchial carcinoma. Accurate anatomical localisation requires further imaging – a lateral CXR or CT scan. CT scanning has the advantage of giving staging information, which is useful in giving accurate prognostic information to the patient. More peripheral lesions like these are less likely to be seen at bronchoscopy compared to the more central tumours shown previously in the book. Therefore, a CT scan with simultaneous biopsy would be most beneficial.

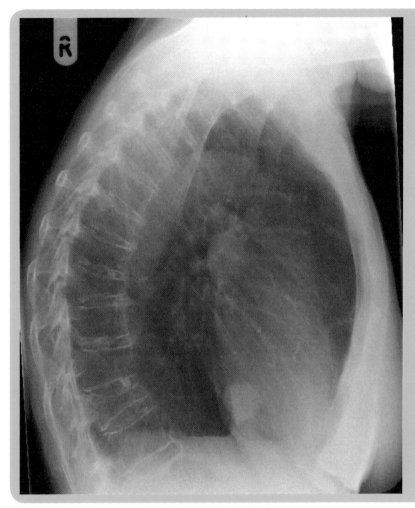

Q: The following are complications of inhaled corticosteroid use **except**:

1. Diabetes Mellitus
2. Adrenal suppression
3. Community acquired pneumonia
4. Osteoporosis
5. Oral thrush

THIS CXR SHOWS

This is the lateral film to accompany the PA film [58]. It confirms the mass is located in the RML. Osteoporotic vertebrae with a number of crush fractures are also seen.

CLINICAL INTERPRETATION

These fractures explain the chronic back pain. Osteoporosis is common in post menopausal women particularly in those with chronic illness, such as COPD. Patients with moderate to severe COPD also receive regular high dose inhaled corticosteroid[1], and high dose oral steroids during exacerbations – both are risk factors for the development of osteoporosis.

Inhaled corticosteroids are also associated with an increased risk of pneumonia and are associated with adrenal suppression.[2]

[1] Lancet. 2000; 22;355(9213):1399-403.

[2] Am J Respir Crit Care Med. 2004 1;170(9):960-6.

Q: Which of the following antibiotics are **not** first line in the treatment of non tuberculous mycobacterium?

1. Isoniazid
2. Rifampicin
3. Ethambutol
4. Clarithromycin
5. Ciprofloxacin

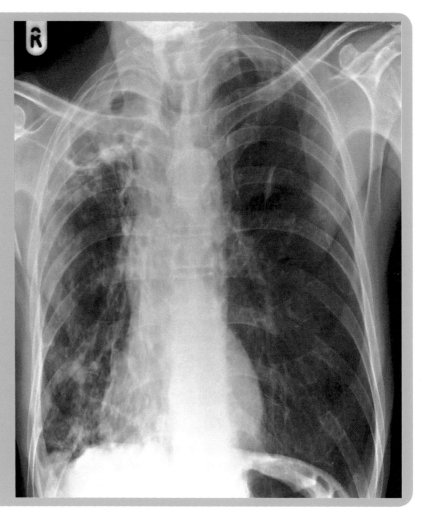

THIS CXR SHOWS

Projection: PA, well centred, well penetrated. Left costophrenic angle not visualised.

Volume loss and fibrotic changes with cavitation in the RUZ suggestive of old TB. There is patchy calcified opacification in the RLZ again possibly due to old TB. Left lung is hyperinflated but relatively spared

CLINICAL INTERPRETATION

Non-tuberculous mycobacteria include *mycobacterium Malmoense, mycobacterium Kansasii* and *mycobacterium Xenoptii*. These organisms are not usually highly pathogenic and cause secondary infection only in patients with pre-existing lung disease (often caused by *mycobacterium tuberculosis* or interstitial lung disease). In this case *mycobacterium malmoense* was isolated from two different specimens and in view of her worsening clinical symptoms she received 2 years of anti-mycobacterial chemotherapy.

[1] Clarithromycin vs ciprofloxacin as adjuncts to rifampicin and ethambutol in treating opportunist mycobacterial lung diseases and an assessment of *Mycobacterium vaccae* immunotherapy *Thorax* 2008;63:627-634

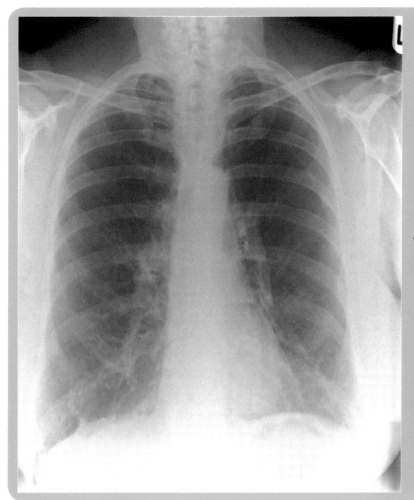

Q: Which of the following investigations would be most useful in this lady?

1. D-dimer assay

2. C-Reactive protein

3. Ventilation perfusion scintigraphy

4. CT pulmonary angiogram

5. Left leg ultrasound

THIS CXR SHOWS

Projection: PA, well centred, under penetrated, adequate field of view.

The pulmonary vessels are prominent. There is tethering of the right hemidiaphragm and paucity of lung markings in both upper zones.

CLINICAL INTERPRETATION

This lady suffers from emphysema and has had lung volume reduction surgery in the past. The CXR is unchanged when compared to the film a few months ago and was requested in view of her profound breathlessness.

The suspicion of DVT and PE could be confirmed with left leg ultrasound. If this confirms DVT, further imaging is unnecessary as it would not alter treatment (therapeutic anticoagulation). V/Q scanning is inappropriate in patients with chronic lung disease with an abnormal chest x-ray,

Q : Which of the following is **not** a cause of hoarseness?

1. Inhaled corticosteroids
2. Professional singing
3. RUL bronchial carcinoma
4. Laryngeal carcinoma
5. Gastro-oesophageal reflux disease (GORD)

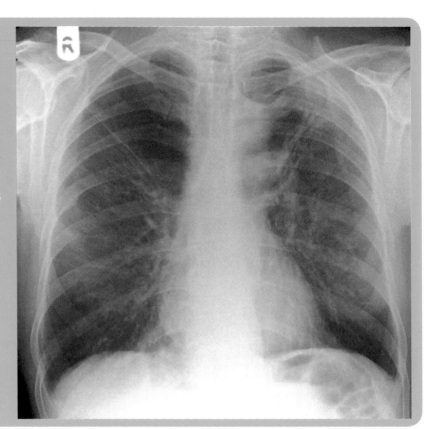

THIS CXR SHOWS

Projection: PA, well centred, well penetrated, adequate field of view.

Old healed right posterior 6th rib fracture. Lateral LUZ streaky opacification extending from the left hilum. Lung hyperinflation

CLINICAL INTERPRETATION

The initial suspicion would be of a pulmonary neoplasm causing left recurrent laryngeal nerve palsy. However, review of previous films showed the abnormality was old.

Unfortunately however, in view of her ear discomfort she was referred to the ENT surgeons who discovered a head and neck neoplasm.

Only left sided bronchial tumours can cause laryngeal nerve palsy as the right recurrent laryngeal nerve does not pass low enough to be involved by most right sided tumours.

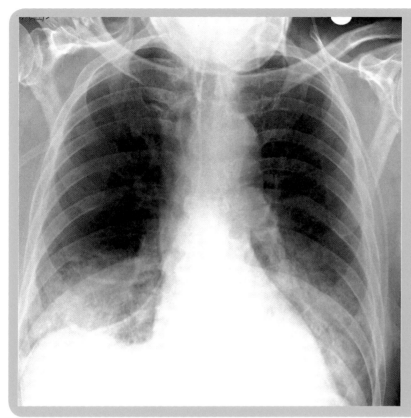

Q: This chest x-ray shows

1. Adult respiratory distress syndrome

2. Acute interstitial pneumonitis (AIP)

3. Left hilar bronchial carcinoma

4. Emphysema and right lower lobe pneumonia

5. Iatrogenic pneumonia

THIS CXR SHOWS

Projection: PA, well centred, over penetrated, adequate field of view.

There is bilateral patchy consolidation in this under-penetrated plain film.

There is a nasogastric feeding tube in the right lower lobe bronchus.

CLINICAL INTERPRETATION

Having made a good recovery from his left sided pneumonia, this man was sent from ICU to HDU with a nasogastric feeding tube in situ. The position of the tube was "confirmed clinically" and feeding was commenced. When his condition deteriorated, this CXR was requested. The NG tube is clearly in the right lower lobe bronchus; the feed has caused a chemical pneumonitis, and secondary bacterial pneumonia.

Recognising the correct location of nasogastric tubes and central intravenous catheters is an essential skill for all practicing clinicians.

Q : Which of the following symptoms did he present with?

1. Erythema nodosum

2. Macroscopic haematuria

3. Pleuritic chest pain

4. Melaena

5. Rash

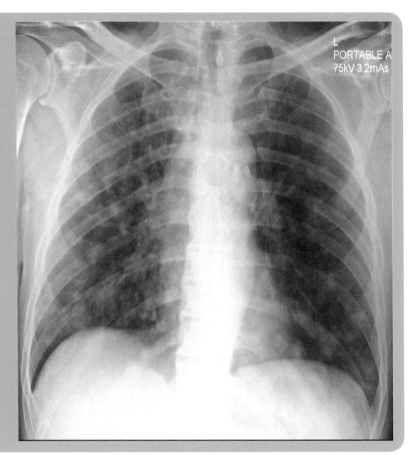

THIS CXR SHOWS

Projection: Portable AP, well centred, well penetrated, adequate field of view.

Large nodular opacities seen throughout both lung fields.

CLINICAL INTERPRETATION

The history and X-ray appearances strongly suggest a malignant process. The multiple metastases in the lungs are suggestive of a renal cell carcinoma when accounting for the patient's renal tract symptoms. As symptoms from the renal tract are often mild and insidious, or may be ignored by the patient the presenting symptoms are frequently secondary to metastatic spread, in this case the systemic effects of disseminated malignancy.

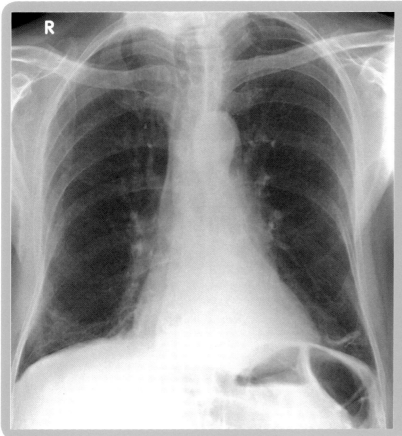

Q : Which of the following features would suggest underlying bronchiectasis?

1. Positive cANCA

2. Upper zone nodular shadowing

3. Pleural calcification

4. Recurrent pleural effusions

5. Chronic sputum production

THIS CXR SHOWS

Projection: PA, well centred, adequately penetrated, adequate field of view.

There is left basal atelectasis and right lower zone streaky opacification

CLINICAL INTERPRETATION

The right basal changes are consistent with recent right lower lobe pneumonia. The left basal atelectasis may represent previous pneumonia.

Recurrent pneumonic episodes can be explained by bronchiectasis, which is often associated with minor changes, or indeed a normal CXR. HRCT is the investigation of choice: in this case there was moderate bronchiectasis bilaterally.

Q: Which of the following would be the most appropriate therapy?

1. Intravenous pamidronate
2. Palliative radiotherapy
3. Radical radiotherapy
4. Left pneumonectomy
5. Surgical debulking

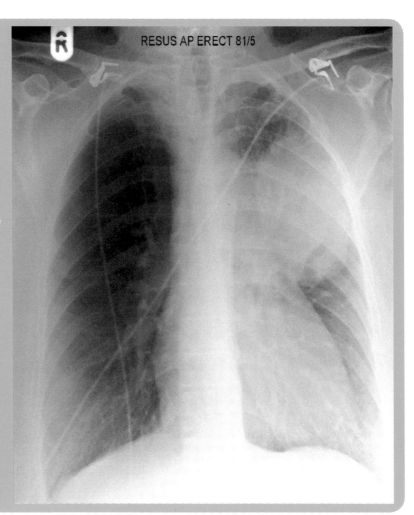

RESUS AP ERECT 81/5

THIS CXR SHOWS

Projection: AP, well centred, well penetrated, adequate field of view.

There is a 10 cm mass in the LUL causing volume loss.

CLINICAL INTERPRETATION

This lady presented to the ENT department with hoarseness of the voice. Direct laryngoscopy revealed a left vocal cord palsy. Left recurrent laryngeal nerve palsy can be caused by compression of the nerve at any point through its course, in this case by a large lung mass.

Recurrent laryngeal nerve palsy is a poor prognostic indicator in lung cancer as it suggests mediastinal involvement, and hence T4 disease. T4, inoperable disease includes mediastinal organ involvement, SVCO, vertebral body involvement, malignant pleural or pericardial effusion and satellite nodule within the same lobe as the primary tumour

Answer: 2) Palliative Radiotherapy ★ ★

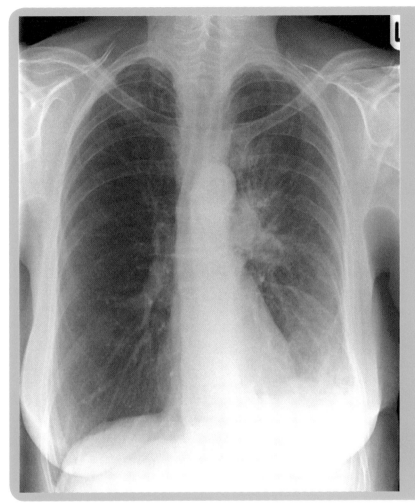

Q: Which investigation is most likely to give you a histological diagnosis?

1. Bronchoscopy

2. Thoracocentesis

3. CT guided lung biopsy

4. Ultrasound guided pleural biopsy

5. Sputum cytology

THIS CXR SHOWS

Projection: PA, well centred, well penetrated, adequate field of view.

There is a left sided pleural effusion of at least moderate size

There is a 3 cm x 3 cm irregular soft tissue opacity projecting just behind the left hilum.

CLINICAL INTERPRETATION

This film is suggestive of advanced bronchial malignancy. Diagnostic approaches are: sputum cytology, which is poorly sensitive; pleural aspiration; and bronchoscopy, as the tumour appears to be central. Bronchoscopy is always the investigation of choice in patients with lung carcinoma and haemoptysis. Pleural fluid cytology has a lower sensitivity than bronchoscopy.

Malignant pleural effusion is a poor prognostic sign: it signifies pleural metastases, and therefore stage IV disease. Prognosis without treatment is in the order of weeks to months.

Q: What is the minimum volume of pleural fluid required to be visible on a lateral chest x-ray?

1. 10ml
2. 50ml
3. 100ml
4. 200ml
5. 500ml

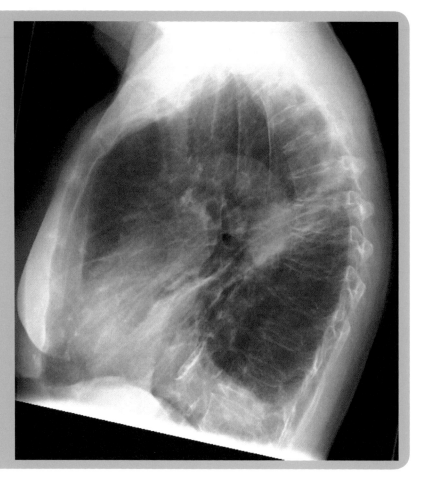

THIS CXR SHOWS

This lateral film reveals a mass in the apical segment of the LLL and a left sided pleural effusion.

CLINICAL INTERPRETATION

This is the left lateral view of the same patient [Case 67] indicating the use of lateral films in this type of case. If no endobronchial lesion is seen at bronchoscopy the apical segment of the LLL should be targeted.

The use of lateral chest x-rays have now largely been superseded by CT scanning but time constraints may not allow CT scanning prior to bronchoscopy. In these cases a lateral film can be most helpful.

50ml is the minimum volume required to visualise on lateral x-ray compared to 200ml for a plain PA radiograph.[1]

[1] Br Med Bull. 2005; 14;72:31-47.

Answer: 2) 50ml

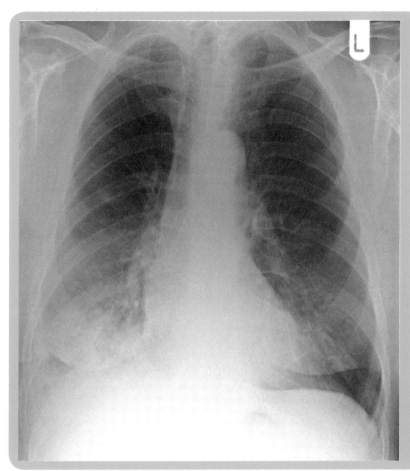

Q : Which of the following features is **not** evident on this chest x-ray?

1. Right lower lobe consolidation

2. Tracheal deviation

3. Left Hilar lymphadenopathy

4. Cardiomegaly

5. Right sided volume loss

THIS CXR SHOWS

Projection: PA, well centred, under penetrated, adequate field of view.

The heart is borderline enlarged. There is pulmonary congestion. There is also dense heterogenous opacification in the RLZ with deviation of the trachea to the right, suggesting right sided volume loss.

CLINICAL INTERPRETATION

This man has heart failure with superadded pneumonia. The treatment of heart failure revolves around fluid restriction and the use of diuretics, however patients with pneumonia are frequently fluid deplete, with or without acute renal impairment. Careful normalisation of physiological parameters is the cornerstone of management of such complex cases; invasive monitoring and a high dependency environment may be required.

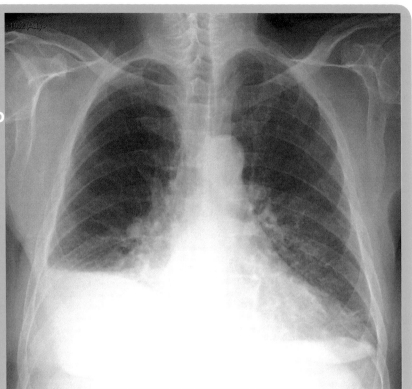

Q : What investigation would you like to perform?

1. Pleural aspiration
2. Echocardiogram
3. Myocardial perfusion scan
4. CT pulmonary angiogram
5. Serum Troponin

THIS CXR SHOWS

Projection: PA, well centred, adequate penetration, adequate field of view.

Cardiomegaly. There is right basal consolidation, and a right sided pleural effusion of at least moderate size.

CLINICAL INTERPRETATION

This is the same patient as case [69]. This repeat CXR confirmed worsening of the RLZ changes and there is now a moderately sized pleural effusion. Aspiration revealed pus in the intrapleural space. Failure to respond to antibiotic therapy, swinging fevers, and development of pleural effusion should increase clinical suspicion of empyema. Treatment is by intercostal drainage, and prolonged antibiotic therapy.

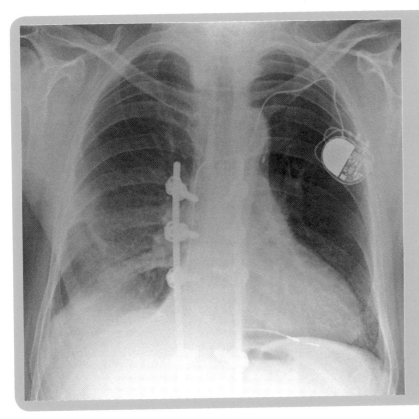

Q: What is the next most appropriate measure?

1. Give Fresh frozen plasma

2. Give Tranexamic acid

3. Stop warfarin and give 5mg oral vitamin K

4. Stop warfarin and restart when INR <5

5. Stop warfarin and switch to intravenous heparin

THIS CXR SHOWS

Projection: PA, well centred, adequately penetrated, adequate field of view.

Tenting of the right hemidiaphragm with patchy opacification below the horizontal fissure. There is also a permanent pacemaker in the left upper zone, and bilateral Harrington rods in position adjacent to the thoracic spine.

CLINICAL INTERPRETATION

An elevated INR alone can explain haemoptysis, but alternative diagnosis must be sought, particularly in a man of this age. Common causes of haemoptysis include: bronchial malignancy; mycobacterial infection; pneumonia; pulmonary embolus; fungal infection, aspergilloma; arteriovenous malformation; inhaled foreign body; bronchial trauma.

Guidelines recommend in patients with INR >8 and minor bleeding but with risk factors for major bleeding (including the elderly) to stop warfarin and administer 0.5mg intravenous or 5mg oral vitamin K. Warfarin is recommenced when INR <5 if still indicated.[1]

[1] British National Formulary March 2009

Q: Which of the following has not been shown to be associated with lung carcinoma?

1. Tobacco smoke
2. Silicosis
3. Radon Gas
4. Asbestos
5. Alcohol

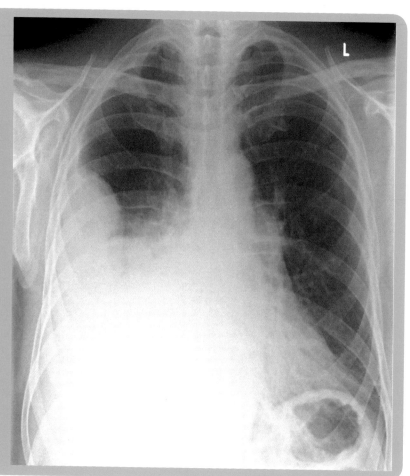

THIS CXR SHOWS

Projection: PA, well centred, adequately penetrated, adequate field of view.

There is a large, round, dense opacity laterally placed in the RLZ. There is an associated pleural effusion. There is also < 1 cm opacity lying between the 2nd and 3rd ribs in the lateral LUZ.

CLINICAL INTERPRETATION

The most likely diagnosis is disseminated bronchial malignancy. The primary tumour is large. There is an associated pleural effusion which is presumably malignant. The lesion in the left upper zone is likely to be a metastasis.

Lung cancer is often slow growing, and onset is insidious: over 80 % of patients present with inoperable disease. Treatment is then palliative, aiming to alleviate symptoms of pain, breathlessness and haemoptysis.

All of the listed factors have been linked to lung cancer with the exception of alcohol.

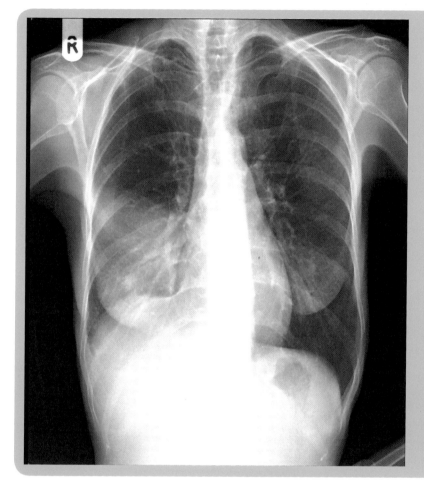

Q: Where is the abnormality?

1. Right lower lobe
2. Right middle lobe
3. Right upper lobe
4. Soft tissue overlying the right mid-zone
5. Right hilar mass

CXR 73b

A throat swab returns a positive PCR result for influenza A. Bronchoscopy was performed due to failure of the abnormality to clear over 4 days.

Q: Which organism did we isolate from bronchoalveolar lavage?

1. Influenza A

2. *Mycoplasma pneumoniae*

3. *Pneumocystis Jirovecii*

4. *Klebsiella Pneumoniae*

5. *Staphylococcus aureus*

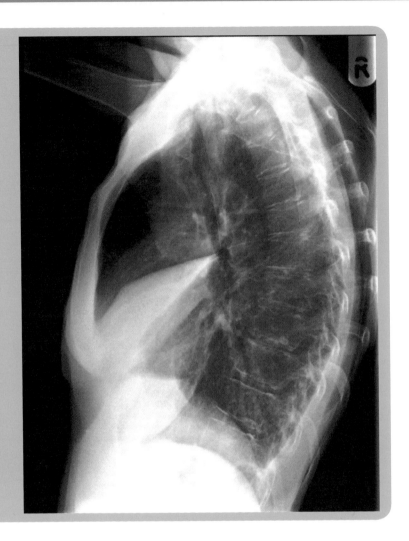

THIS CXR SHOWS

Projection: PA, well centred, adequate penetration, appropriate field of view.

On the PA film there is loss of the right heart border and dense opacification overlying the right lower-mid zone indicating consolidation within the right middle lobe.

This is confirmed on the lateral view.

CLINICAL INTERPRETATION

This lady has community acquired pneumonia, which may follow influenza infection. True viral pneumonia is thought to be relatively rare, although viral pathogens can be frequently isolated by PCR, the clinical significance of this is uncertain.[1]

Mortality during influenza epidemics can be high and is primarily due to secondary bacterial pneumonia. *Staphylococcus aureus* is classically associated with post-influenza pneumonia and empirical anti-staphylococcal coverage should be considered in patients presenting with severe CAP following flu.

[1] Jennings LC et al. Incidence and characteristics of viral community acquired pneumonia in adults . Thorax 2008;63(7):658-9

Answer: 5) Staphylococcus aureus

This 57 year old man presents with breathlessness. His resting arterial gases reveal type 2 respiratory failure.

CXR 74

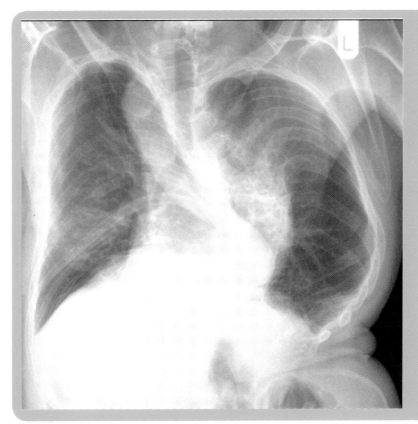

Q : Which treatment offers the best survival benefit?

1. Long Term Oxygen Therapy (LTOT)

2. Thiazide Diuretic

3. Loop Diuretic

4. Ambulatory oxygen cylinders

5. Non Invasive Ventilation (NIV)

THIS CXR SHOWS

Projection: PA, adequate penetration, adequate field of view.

This CXR shows marked chest wall deformity with kyphoscoliosis concave to the left

CLINICAL INTERPRETATION

This patient has marked kyphoscoliosis.

Patients with kyphoscoliosis run the risk of developing respiratory insufficiency due to alveolar hypoventilation. They should be offered respiratory support which aims to improve survival.

Long term oxygen therapy (LTOT) and home non invasive ventilation (NIV) can be offered to such individuals. NIV provides better symptom control by correcting hypercapnia and better survival benefit when compared to LTOT.[1]

[1] Chest. 2006 130(6):1828-33.

Q: The most likely cause of this ladies clubbing is?

1. Type I diabetes mellitus

2. Multiple endocrine neoplasia type II

3. Transposition of the great arteries

4. Atrial myxoma and pulmonary fibrosis

5. Bronchiectasis

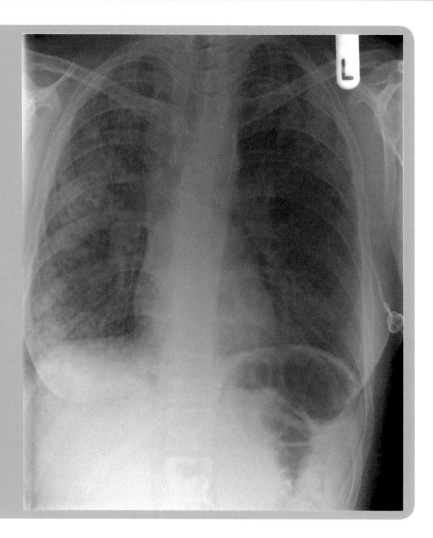

THIS CXR SHOWS

Projection: PA, right rotation, well penetrated, inadequate field of view as right costophrenic angle not visualised.

There is patchy opacification with air bronchograms throughout the right lung and the LUZ.

There are small ring shadows throughout both lungs. There is a left sided venous "Portacath" device.

CLINICAL INTERPRETATION

The diagnosis is Cystic Fibrosis. The CXR shows cysts throughout both lung fields, widespread airspace opacification due to current infection, and a long term venous access device to allow repeated intravenous antibiotic therapy.

Remember that investigations can only narrow your clinical suspicion, the clinical details give the differential diagnosis. How many causes of clubbing and hyper-glycaemia are there in a 19 year old girl?

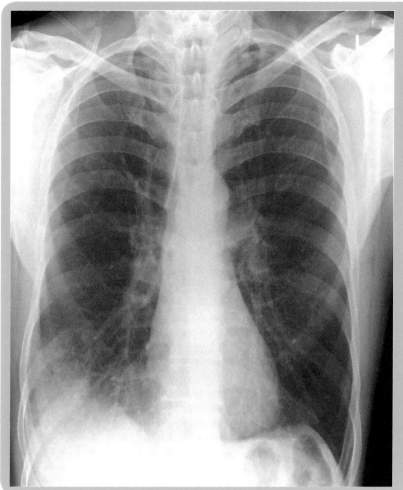

Q : Which antibiotics would you include in his management

1. Intravenous macrolide

2. Intravenous quinolone

3. Rifampicin and Flucloxacillin

4. Oral vancomycin

5. Intravenous metronidazole

THIS CXR SHOWS

Projection: PA, well centred, well penetrated, adequate field of view.

There is patchy opacification in the RLL, obliterating the right hemi-diaphragm. There is oxygen tubing overlying the right lung field.

CLINICAL INTERPRETATION

Basal consolidation in the presence of an abnormal swallow reflex should rise the suspicion of aspiration pneumonia. The trachea is curved slightly to the right, and the right main bronchus branches at a less acute angle than the left main bronchus – these anatomical traits lead aspirated foodstuffs to tend to pass into the right basal segments, rather than the left. Treatment should cover aerobic and anaerobic pathogens, and the cause of the defective swallow should be elucidated.

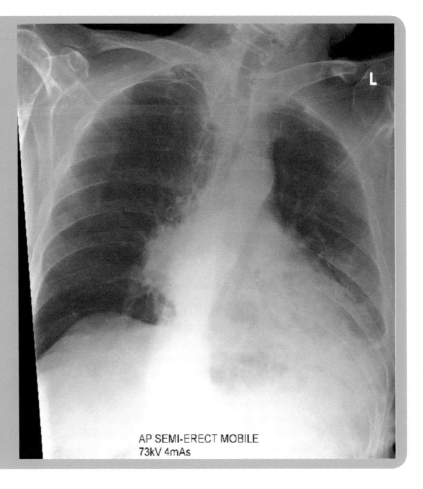

Q : This X-ray shows

1. Lung carcinoma

2. Right ventricular hypertrophy

3. Right pleural effusion

4. Adequate field of view

5. Possible mediastinal pathology

AP SEMI-ERECT MOBILE
73kV 4mAs

THIS CXR SHOWS

Projection: Technically poor film. AP semi erect, off centre and rotated to the right, under penetrated, inadequate field of view as right costophrenic sulcus is missing from view.

The right hilum is bulky despite the technical faults of the film. The left diaphragm is indistinct.

CLINICAL INTERPRETATION

When no clinical details are available, interpretation of the chest X-ray can be difficult. The apparent bulky right hilum could be entirely factitious, due to projection errors, or a large right hilar tumour. There is the suspicion of LLL consolidation, but again this could be due to projection. Assessing the mediastinum is particularly challenging on grossly rotated films and interpretation should be under taken with caution.

This is a common clinical problem – the best guess is frequently the best we can offer.

This 54 year old man has chest pain, palpitations and light headedness. His ECG confirms atrial fibrillation.

CXR 78

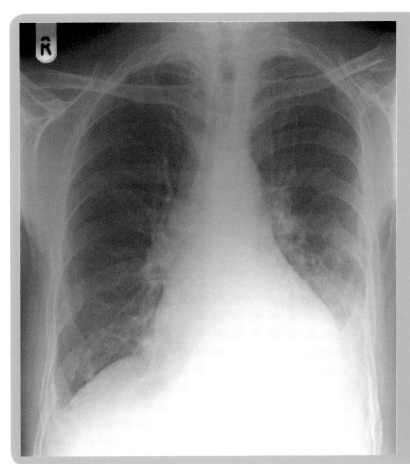

Q: Which of the following may be considered **inappropriate** in this case?

1. Digoxin
2. Amiodarone
3. Metoprolol
4. Aspirin
5. Warfarin

THIS CXR SHOWS

Projection: PA, well centred, under penetrated, adequate field of view.

There are multiple old left rib fractures. Increased cardiothoracic ratio.

Dense left basal opacification.

CLINICAL INTERPRETATION

Left sided basal pneumonia, cardiomegaly and previous rib fractures in a man with atrial fibrillation.

The commonest causes of atrial fibrillation in the UK are: ischaemic heart disease; valvular heart disease; hypertensive heart disease; pneumonia; and alcohol excess. The clue here is the rib fractures – this patient was a chronic abuser of alcohol.

Q : The X-ray shows:

1. Bilateral pleural effusions and right volume loss

2. Right pleural thickening and pleural plaques

3. Right upper lobectomy and left hilar mass

4. Pulmonary hypertension and right pleural effusion

5. Bilateral pneumonia and left hilar mass

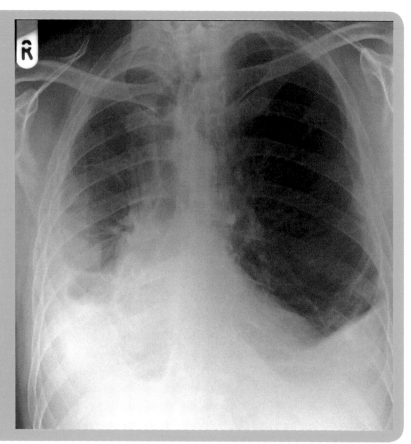

THIS CXR SHOWS

Projection: PA, well centred, well penetrated, adequate field of view.

There is bilateral pleural effusion with loss of volume and collapse of the right lung.

CLINICAL INTERPRETATION

Bilateral pleural effusions suggest: cardiac failure; hypoalbuminaemic state; disseminated malignancy; or bilateral pulmonary disease. The differential is narrowed by pleural aspiration – exudative and transudative effusions have differing aetiologies.

The loss of volume in the right lung, in association with bilateral effusions may represent primary lung tumour with disseminated pleural metastases. A thoracic CT will give more information.

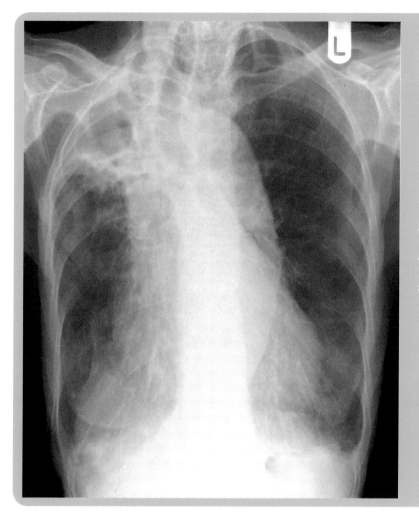

Q: The following features are present except:

1. Hyperinflation
2. Right pleural effusion
3. Unfolding of the aorta
4. Right apical volume loss
5. Mediastinal shift

THIS CXR SHOWS

Projection: PA, well centred, adequate penetration, adequate field of view.

There is unfolding of a dilated thoracic aorta. There is right apical pleural thickening with cavitation

CLINICAL INTERPRETATION

The right apical changes are entirely consistent with mycobacterial infection, however, given the presentation, there may be acute pulmonary infection.

Radiologists will frequently tell you, old x-rays are the most valuable resource in interpreting changes on CXRs, and in this case, the changes were long standing, and an alternative diagnosis was sought.

Q: The following features suggest pulmonary oedema **except**:

1. Kerley B Lines

2. Left atrial enlargement

3. Upper lobe venous diversion

4. Perihilar alveolar shadowing

5. Bilateral pleural effusions

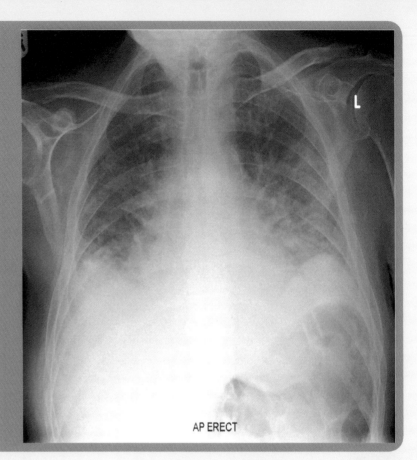

THIS CXR SHOWS

Projection: AP, well centred, under penetrated, adequate field of view but under inspired plain film.

There is cardiomegaly and perihilar congestion – the so called "Bats-wing shadowing"

There is upper lobe venous distension but no Kerley B lines visible.

CLINICAL INTERPRETATION

Although this patient didn't give a history, his distress, sweating, tachypnoea, tachycardia and the fact that he preferred to sit upright was diagnostic of acute pulmonary oedema for which the CXR and ECG (LBBB) were confirmatory. It was an acute event with significantly raised troponin assay and he responded well to oxygen, diuretics, nitrate infusion and opiates.

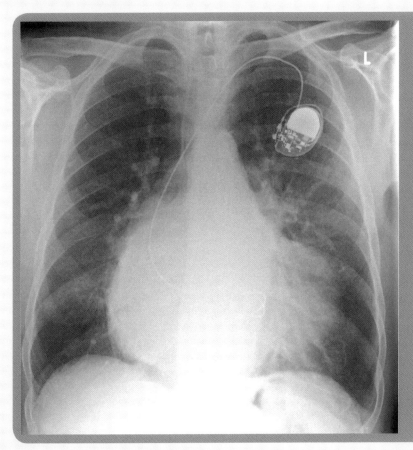

Q : Which of the following is present on this chest x-ray?

1. Dual chamber pacemaker

2. Mechanical aortic valve

3. Subclavian venous line

4. Right clavicle fracture

5. Right ventricular enlargement

THIS CXR SHOWS

Projection: PA, slightly rotated to the left, under penetrated, adequate field of view.

Grossly enlarged right ventricle. There is a mechanical mitral valve *in situ*. There is a single lead ventricular pacemaker.

CLINICAL INTERPRETATION

The most striking finding is gross right ventricular enlargement – the gross leg oedema is due to right ventricular dysfunction. CXR is not an accurate assessment tool for cardiac function however gross cardiomegaly such as this is highly suggestive of ventricular dysfunction.

Echocardiography gives a more accurate functional assessment.

Q: What is the most likely cause of this patients chest pain?

1. Rib fractures

2. Angina

3. Right sided bronchial carcinoma

4. 2cm right apical pneumothorax

5. Pericarditis

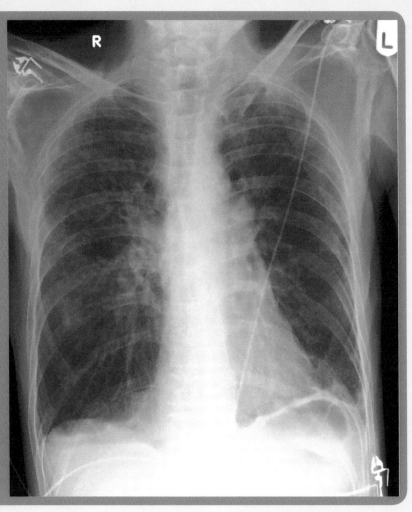

THIS CXR SHOWS

Projection: PA, left rotation, well penetrated, adequate field of view.

There is a fractured posterior right 4th rib but no pneumothorax. The lungs are hyperinflated with streaky fibrotic opacification in the upper zones. There is a 1 cm soft tissue nodule overlying the right 9th posterior rib.

CLINICAL INTERPRETATION

The clinical suspicion here is of rib fracture, which the CXR confirms. However the unexpected finding of a 1 cm diameter lung lesion is of more significance, and may represent a primary lung cancer.

CXR is not indicated to confirm rib fractures – not all fractures are visible on plain film, and confirmation does not change management. The CXR *is* indicated to rule out pneumothorax in cases of trauma, and care should be taken to pick up any unexpected finding, as in this case.

Answer: 1) Rib Fractures

★ ★

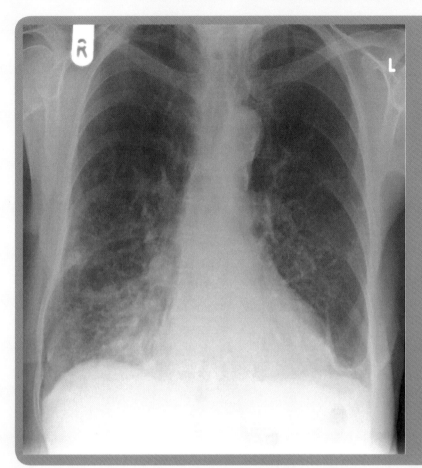

Q: What is the most likely causative pathogen?

1. *Haemophilus influenzae*

2. *Moraxella Catarrhalis*

3. *Campylobacter Jejuni*i

4. *Streptococcus Pneumoniae*

5. *Pseudomonas Aeruginosa*

THIS CXR SHOWS

Projection: PA, well centred, well penetrated, adequate field of view.

There is RMZ consolidation and a large bulla in the LLL. There are emphysematous changes in the upper zones.

CLINICAL INTERPRETATION

This film shows a right sided pneumonia in a patient with established COPD.

Haemophilus influenzae, moraxella catarrhalis and *pseudomonas species* are all more frequent causes of CAP in patients with COPD, however, *streptococcus pneumoniae* remains the major causative organism.

Proximal obstruction by tumour should always be considered in anyone with a smoking history, so a 4–6 week interval CXR should be requested. If the changes do not resolve, CT and bronchoscopy are indicated.

Q : Which of the following terms is used to describe this appearance?

1. Honey combing
2. Cavitatory
3. Nodular
4. Oedematous
5. Plaque

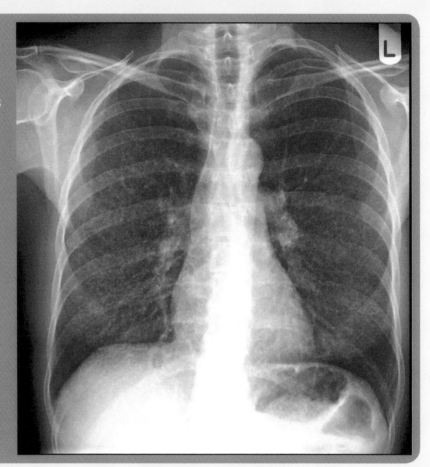

THIS CXR SHOWS

Projection: PA, Technically adequate

There is bilateral, diffuse nodularity to the lungs in an almost miliary type pattern.

CLINICAL INTERPRETATION

This middle aged woman had a diagnosis of sarcoidosis.

Diffuse nodularity on plain CXR carries a differential of benign and malignant disorders. The first step would be to compare with any previous plain films. If these are not available or there is evidence of radiological progression on the most recent film, further detailed imaging with CT is required and lung tissue should be obtained.

Clinical features, past medical problems and a detailed occupational, recreational and medication history can often provide clues in cases of interstitial lung disease.

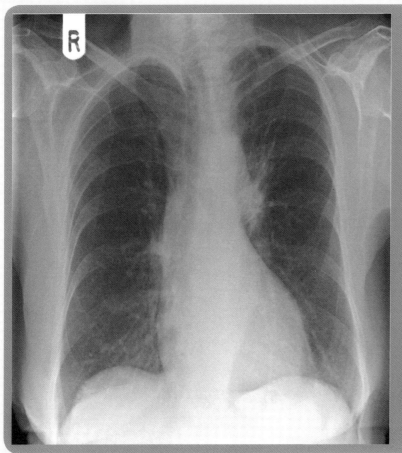

Q : Which blood test is likely to be **most** useful from the following?

1. Serum Angiotensin converting enzyme

2. D-dimer assay

3. Serum Calcium

4. CA-19-9

5. Prostate specific antigen (PSA)

THIS CXR SHOWS

Projection: PA, well centred, well penetrated, adequate field of view.

Scoliosis convex to the left. There is a spiculated left hilar mass extending into LUL.

There is also a small granuloma in right upper lobe secondary to previous TB.

CLINICAL INTERPRETATION

Constipation is common in the elderly, with a wide differential. In the context of a CXR suspicious of lung cancer, the serum calcium level should be checked. Squamous cell carcinoma of the lung can release parathyroid related peptide, leading to increased calcium release from bone. Hypercalcaemia can also be a consequence of bone metastases. Hypercalcaemia causes abdominal pain secondary to constipation, renal tract calculi and bowel spasm, and can cause psychological symptoms, most frequently confusion.

CXR 87

This 71 year old man presents with weight loss and fever. Pleural fluid sampling is performed

Q: What micro-organism is most likely to be isolated from the pleural fluid?

1. *Streptococcus pneumoniae*

2. *Streptococcus Milleri*

3. *Streptococcus viridans*

4. *Mycoplasma pneumoniae*

5. Pseudomonas species.

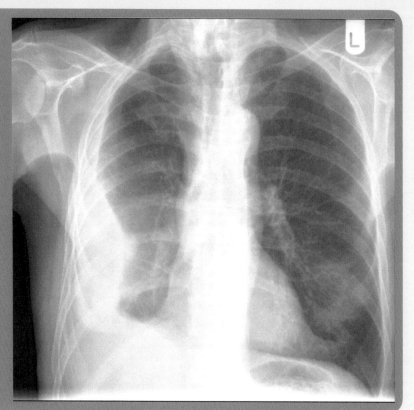

THIS CXR SHOWS

Projection: PA, well centred, well penetrated, adequate field of view.

There is a peripheral D-shaped opacity in the right lung field consistent with a loculated pleural effusion.

There is a pulmonary nodule in the right mid-zone. The left lung field is clear.

CLINICAL INTERPRETATION

The D-shaped pleural effusion is classical of empyema, although this appearance can also be seen with pleural thickening or other causes of a loculated pleural effusion.

The nodule in the right mid-zone raises suspicion of a malignant effusion. Secondary infection of a malignant effusion may follow pleural instrumentation such as pleural aspiration, intercostal drainage or thoracoscopy.

The most common organism isolated from empyema in the UK is currently *Streptococcus milleri* group.[1,2]

[1] Maskell NA, *et al.* UK controlled trial of intrapleural streptokinase for pleural infection. *N Engl J Med*. 2005;352:865-874.

[2] Chalmers JD et al, Risk factors for complicated parapneumonic effusion and empyema on presentation to hospital with community acquired pneumonia. *Thorax* 2009; 64:592-597

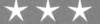

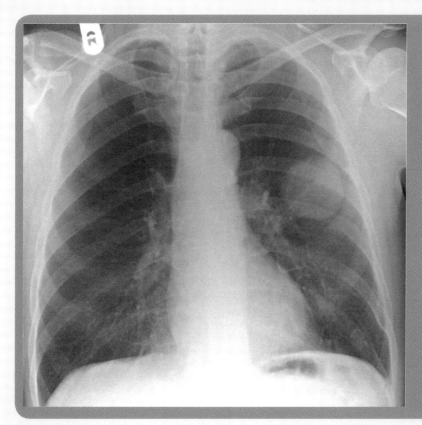

Q: The most likely cause of this mans seizure is:

1. Cerebrovascular disease
2. Glioma
3. Cerebral metastases
4. Hypercalcaemia
5. Alcohol withdrawal

THIS CXR SHOWS

Projection: PA, well centred, well penetrated, adequate field of view.

There is a LMZ 6cm opacity of regular outline and uniform density.

CLINICAL INTERPRETATION

A seizure in an elderly man is unlikely to be due to primary epilepsy. Causes of secondary seizure are: space occupying lesion, either primary brain tumour, or secondary deposit; intracerebral haemorrhage; stroke; venous sinus thrombosis; meningo-encephalitis. Common things being common, the most likely diagnosis is a metastatic deposit in the brain, secondary to lung cancer. The differential of a round lesion on a CXR is: carcinoma; secondary tumour; abscess; encysted interlobar effusion; hydatid cyst; AV malformation; carcinoid; aspergilloma; rheumatoid nodule; hamartoma and bronchogenic cyst.

Q: This x-ray shows the following abnormalities except:

1. Old rib fractures
2. Aortic calcification
3. RMZ consolidation
4. Left fractured clavicle
5. LMZ consolidation

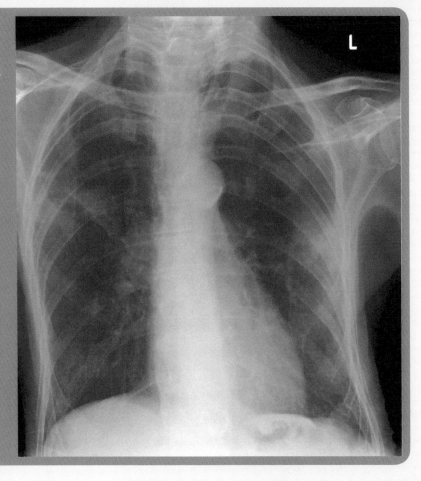

THIS CXR SHOWS

Projection: PA, well centred, well penetrated, adequate field of view.

There are multiple rib fractures and multiple, scattered areas of patchy opacification, mainly in the right upper and the left lateral mid zones.

CLINICAL INTERPRETATION

Multiple previous rib fractures suggests gait disturbance, or alcohol abuse. Upper zone opacification is compatible with mycobacterial infection. To make an accurate diagnosis of mycobacterial infection sputum or bronchial washings obtained at bronchoscopy must be cultured for 6 weeks.

In this case the CXR changes were longstanding, and sputum culture negative. The cough was again a longstanding issue. Remember that old CXRs are invaluable, as not all changes are new.

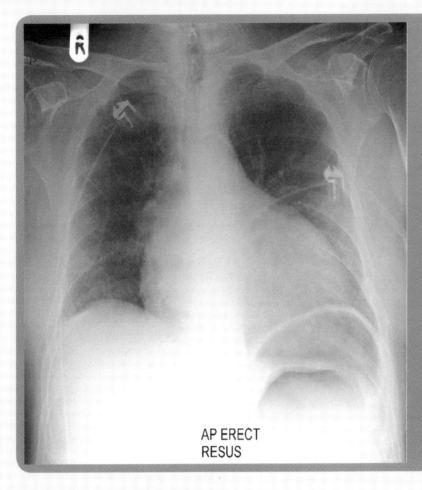

AP ERECT
RESUS

Q : Which of the following is required?

1. Echocardiogram

2. Laparotomy

3. CT aortogram

4. CT pulmonary angiogram

5. Upper GI endoscopy

THIS CXR SHOWS

Projection: AP semi erect, well centred, under penetrated.

The heart is enlarged. There is evidence of free gas under the left hemidiaphragm.

CLINICAL INTERPRETATION

There should be no free air under the diaphragm – its presence indicates a perforated abdominal viscous. Causes of bowel perforation include: peptic ulceration, usually duodenal; Crohn's disease; diverticular disease; ulcerative colitis; and malignancy.

Patients with free air in the peritoneal space require urgent investigation to elucidate the cause – referral to a surgical team, CT scanning, and consideration of laparotomy, or laparoscopy.

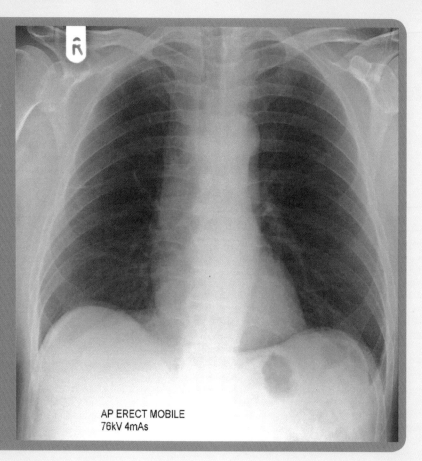

Q: Which of the following may be the cause of this patients fatigue?

1. Myasthenia gravis
2. Radiotherapy
3. Left hilar bronchogenic carcinoma
4. Hypothyroidism
5. Left ventricular failure

AP ERECT MOBILE
76kV 4mAs

THIS CXR SHOWS

Projection: AP, well centred, well penetrated, adequate field of view.

The upper right mediastinum is enlarged

CLINICAL INTERPRETATION

The upper mediastinal enlargement is due to a thymoma – this tumour is associated with adult onset myasthenia gravis, the cause of his fatigue. The mediastinum consists of: the heart; the great vessels; oesophagus; trachea; phrenic and cardiac nerves; thoracic duct; thymus, or it's remnant; and lymph nodes. Enlargement of any of these structures can cause radiological enlargement of the mediastinum.

Distinction between the causes of mediastinal enlargement is not usually possible on plain film; a CT of the thorax is advised.

Answer: 1) Myasthenia Gravis ★ ★

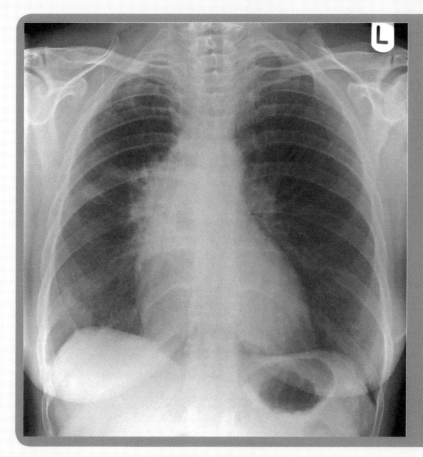

Q : The following are considered oncological emergencies **except:**

1. Spinal cord compression
2. Superior vena cava obstruction
3. Tumour lysis syndrome
4. Neutropenic sepsis
5. Obstructive jaundice

THIS CXR SHOWS

Projection: PA, well centred, well penetrated, adequate field of view.

There is a dense, irregular right hilar opacity. A superior vena caval stent is seen crossing the right hilum. There are calcified opacities in the RUZ.

CLINICAL INTERPRETATION

The primary diagnosis is right hilar bronchogenic carcinoma complicated by superior vena caval obstruction. Presentation of SVC obstruction is with: plethora of the face; headache; elevated, non pulsatile JVP; and dilated superficial veins in the distribution of the SVC. Immediate treatment is insertion of a radiologically guided, percutaneous, trans-venous stent to the SVC. Superior vena caval obstruction is frequently the presenting sign of advanced lung cancer. It is a life threatening complication, and should not be missed.

Q: What is the likelihood of recurrent pleural effusion following talc pleurodesis?

1. 5%
2. 10%
3. 30%
4. 50%
5. 80%

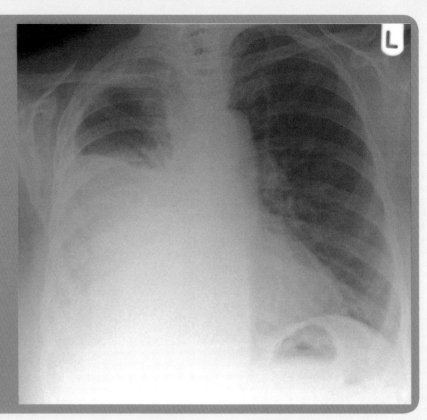

THIS CXR SHOWS

Projection: PA, well centred, under penetrated, adequate field of view.

There is loss of volume in the right lung with dense opacification occupying the RMZ and RLZ. Lung tissue is visible through the opacification, particularly laterally.

CLINICAL INTERPRETATION

Malignant pleural effusion represents pleural metastases, and inoperable disease, with a poor prognosis. Therapy is palliative; either recurrent pleural aspiration, or pleurodesis. The success rate with talc pleurodesis, via intercostal chest drain, is in the range of 80–90%; in the remainder of cases loculated effusions may recur.[1] As the talc is radio-lucent, and causes a radio lucent inflammatory reaction in the pleura, chest x-ray appearances after successful pleurodesis are similar to those of an effusion. Thoracic ultrasound distinguishes between pleural reaction, and effusion.

[1] Chemical pleurodesis for malignant pleural effusions. *Ann Intern Med* 1994; 120: 56-64

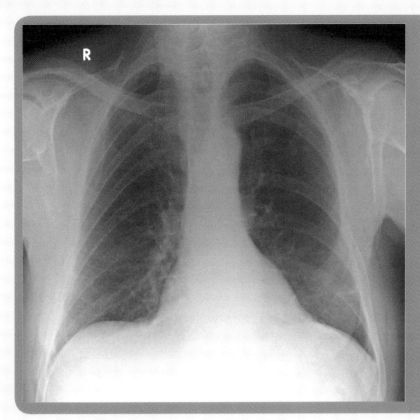

Q: What is the most likely cause of this CXR appearance?

1. Previous surgery
2. Radiotherapy
3. Chemotherapy with opportunistic infection
4. Paget's disease
5. Asbestos exposure

THIS CXR SHOWS

Projection: PA, right rotation, under penetrated, adequate field of view.

The lateral portion of the posterior 6th rib is absent.

There is minor LLZ scarring.

CLINICAL INTERPRETATION

The 6th rib has been removed to improve access to the thoracic cavity during thoracotomy, in this case for left lower lobectomy for metastatic melanoma. The CXR is remarkably normal for a patient who has had half of his left lung removed! The expected finding is of reduced volume of the left lung, however, over time the remaining left upper lobe expands to fill the thoracic cavity. Other features of previous thoracic surgery on a chest x-ray may include midline sternotomy wires.

Q : Which of the following should be considered first?

1. Ultrasound guided pleural aspiration
2. Closed pleural biopsy
3. Commence ACE-Inhibitor therapy
4. Anti-tuberculous chemotherapy
5. Bronchoscopy

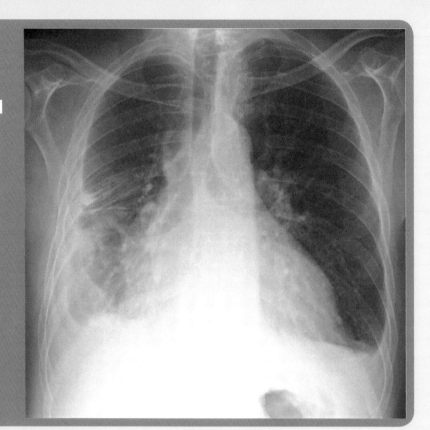

THIS CXR SHOWS

Projection: PA, well centred, well penetrated, adequate field of view.

There is cardiomegaly and bilateral pleural effusions. There is linear scarring emanating from the right pleura, there is also right sided pleural thickening.

CLINICAL INTERPRETATION

Bilateral pleural effusions and cardiomegaly suggest cardiac failure as the cause of this man's lethargy, however cardiac dysfunction cannot explain the right sided pleural changes. Although a single unifying diagnosis is nice for doctors, patients don't read medical textbooks! The pleural changes may be due to active, or old empyema; benign pleural thickening; or malignant mesothelioma. Aspiration of the effusion, ideally under trans-thoracic ultrasound may reveal the diagnosis.

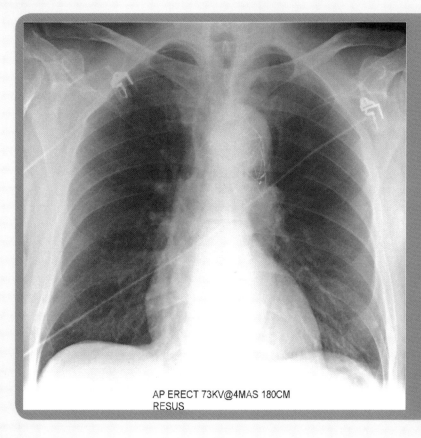

AP ERECT 73KV@4MAS 180CM
RESUS

Q: With what diagnosis did he present?

1. Aortic regurgitation
2. Left sided lung carcinoma
3. Rheumatic mitral valve disease
4. Thoracic aortic aneurysm
5. Thymoma

THIS CXR SHOWS

Projection: AP, well centred, well penetrated, adequate field of view.

There is a stent in the aortic arch, the aorta is unfolded.

CLINICAL INTERPRETATION

This man had a previous thoracic aortic aneurysm, treated with an endovascular stent. Before the advent of endovascular surgery, patients with thoracic aneurysms faced high risk thoracic surgery to repair the defect.

There are no acute changes on this CXR.

Q : The most likely diagnosis is?

1. Right pneumothorax

2. Pulmonary embolism

3. Exacerbation of asthma

4. Acute exacerbation of Chronic obstructive pulmonary disease

5. *Pneumocystic Jirovecii Pneumonia*

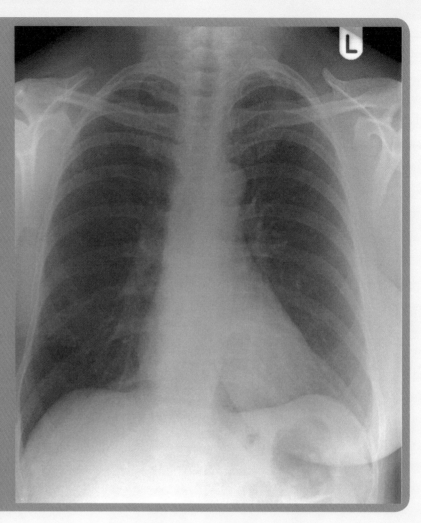

THIS CXR SHOWS

Projection: PA, well centred, well penetrated, adequate field of view.

Previous right mastectomy

CLINICAL INTERPRETATION

The differential diagnosis of acute hypoxaemia in association with normal lung fields on a CXR includes: pulmonary embolus; pulmonary arterial hypertension; pulmonary vasculitis; *pneumocystis jirovecii pneumonia*. A history of malignancy is a major risk factor for venous thromboembolism.

Answer: 2) Pulmonary embolism

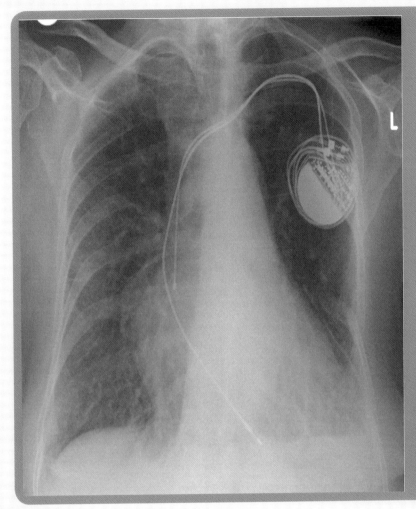

Q: What of the following investigations would be most appropriate initially?

1. Repeat PA chest x-ray
2. Staging CT thorax
3. 24 hour ECG
4. Pacemaker check
5. CT guided lung biopsy

THIS CXR SHOWS

Projection: PA, rotated to the right, well penetrated, adequate field of view.

There is a dual chamber pace maker *in situ* with satisfactory lead position. There is the impression of RUZ medial mediastinal soft tissue round opacity.

CLINICAL INTERPRETATION

This case demonstrates the difficulties of interpreting a poor quality CXR. Although there is a suggestion of a right upper lobe mass, the film is rotated, and on CT scanning the right upper lobe is normal. The CXR does not show any loss of volume of the right lung, as might be expected if the appearances were a tumour - if you are asked to interpret a film such as this, a repeat **PA** CXR may save your patient the radiation associated with a staging CT of the thorax.

In this case, investigating the cause of the collapse takes precedence.

Q: What would be the next most appropriate step in management:

1. Intercostal drain

2. Pleural aspiration

3. Review old chest x-rays and case records

4. Commence continuous positive airways pressure

5. Intravenous diuretics

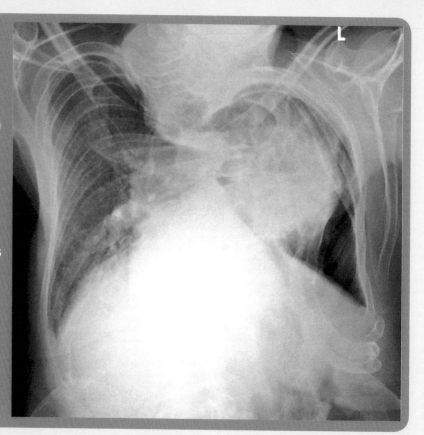

THIS CXR SHOWS

There is gross thoracic scoliosis which impairs assessment of mediastinum and lungs. There is paucity of lung markings in the LMZ – this may represent pneumothorax, or bullae.

CLINICAL INTERPRETATION

Kyphoscoliosis can cause significant respiratory embarrassment, notably alveolar hypoventilation. Patients with kyphoscoliosis may develop type 1, or type 2 respiratory failure. Such patients with chronic type 2 failure are well treated with non-invasive ventilatory support, usually nocturnal. In this case it is important to distinguish between pneumothorax and bulla – pneumothorax is a contra-indication to positive pressure ventilation.

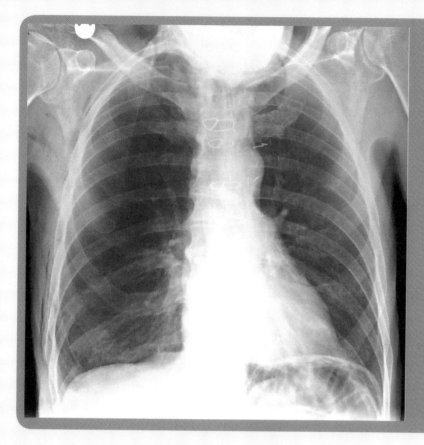

Q : **Which of the following is the most appropriate initial management?**

1. Simple analgesia

2. CT chest and abdomen

3. Intercostal chest drainage

4. Therapeutic pleural aspiration

5. CT brain

THIS CXR SHOWS

Projection: PA, well centred, well penetrated, adequate field of view.

There are fractures of the right 9th and 10th ribs, with overlying surgical emphysema. There is a right apical pneumothorax. Mid-line sternotomy sutures indicate previous cardiac surgery.

CLINICAL INTERPRETATION

The apical traumatic pneumothorax should be treated – current guidelines recommend intercostal drainage. However, this man has dementia, and may not tolerate a chest drain well. Symptomatic treatment in the form of analgesia, and oxygen for hypoxaemia, is a reasonable alternative. Remember that you are treating the patient and not the chest x-ray.

Q : The most likely cause of this abnormality is

1. RML pneumonia
2. Bronchial carcinoma
3. Pulmonary contusion
4. Pulmonary embolism
5. Mycobacterium tuberculosis

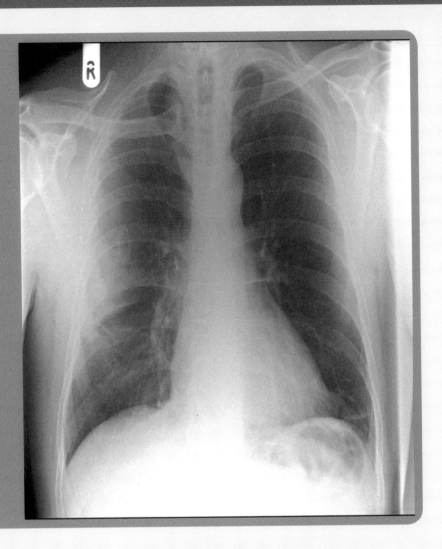

THIS CXR SHOWS

Projection: PA, slight rotated. Adequately inspired and penetrated.

Atelectasis left base.

There is dense, homogenous shadowing in the right mid-zone adjacent to the chest wall.

There is no pneumothorax.

CLINICAL INTERPRETATION

This abnormality is due to traumatic lung contusion. This is a relatively common finding in major trauma. The consequences of less major injuries are often evident on medical wards-always check the chest film for ribs fractures, humerus and clavicular fractures and for small pneumothoraces, all of which may complicate relatively minor trauma, particularly In the elderly.

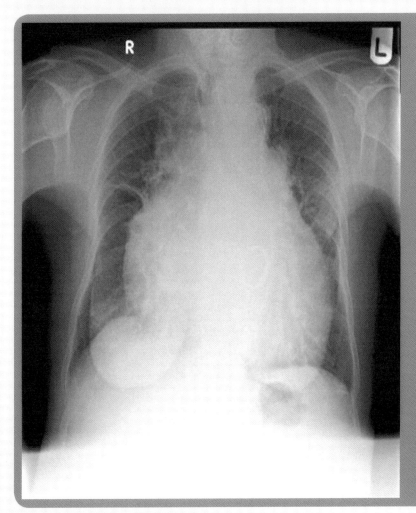

Q: The most likely cause of her syncope is:

1. Myocardial infarction
2. Pulmonary embolism
3. Cardiac arrythmia
4. Aortic valve rupture
5. Community acquired pneumonia

THIS CXR SHOWS

Projection: PA, technically adequate.

Grossly dilated heart. Prosthetic aortic value evident

There is some upper lobe venous diversion and fluffy shadowing suggestive of mild pulmonary oedema.

CLINICAL INTERPRETATION

This elderly lady has massive Enlargement of the cardiac Silhouette affecting all 4 chambers of the heart. The appearances are typical of dilated cardiomyopathy (DCM) About 20-30% of DCM cases are familial. In this age group, more common causes would be toxins (most frequently chronic alcohol abuse but heavy metal poisoning and chemotherapy agents such as doxorubicin give the same presentation. DCM may also complicate connective tissue diseases and HIV infection, or may be the aftermath of viral myocarditis (which may have been asymptomatic).

★ ★

Answer: 3) Cardiac arrhythmia

CXR 103

**This 51 year old man has a history of chronic renal failure.
He is a smoker**

Q: The following features are present on this chest x-ray except:

1. Left upper lobectomy

2. Tunnelled venous line

3. LLL collapse

4. Mediastinal shift

5. Increased bronchovascular markings

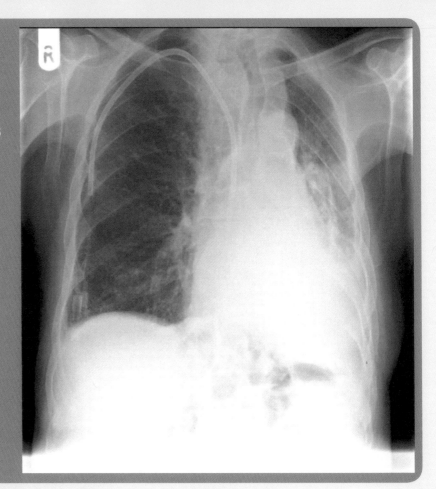

THIS CXR SHOWS

Projection: PA, slight rotated. adequately inspired and penetrated.

There is a tunnelled line with the tip in the superior vena cava.

The left heart border is obliterated and the left costophrenic angle is obscured. There is left lower lobe collapse with movement of the mediastinum to the left and opacity in the left lower zone obscuring the diaphragm.

CLINICAL INTERPRETATION

This gentleman has chronic renal failure and is receiving haemodialysis. This is suggested by the presence of a tunneled venous access line into the superior vena cava.

Chronic renal failure is not a cause of left lower lobe collapse however. In a 51 year old smoker the most likely diagnosis would be an obstructing left lower lobe bronchogenic carcinoma.

Often left lower lobe collapse is more subtle because the left lower lobe collapses medially and posteriorly, the only sign is often an opacity "hidden" behind the heart shadow. This gives the left heart border an unusually straight appearance. The double shadow is referred to as the "sail sign".

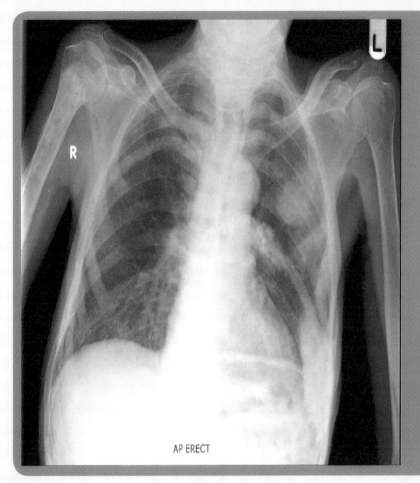

AP ERECT

Q: The most likely cause of this appearance is:

1. Primary hyperparathyroidism
2. Paget's disease
3. Pleural plaques
4. Chronic osteomyelitis
5. Disseminated prostate carcinoma

THIS CXR SHOWS

Projection: AP erect film. The patient is off centre. Adequate penetration and inspiration.

Widespread sclerotic bony metastases infiltrating the right humerus, 4th and 5th right posterior ribs and the 2nd to 5th right anterior ribs. The 7th right posterior rib is also involved.

Raised left hemidiaphragm.

The lung fields are clear although some areas are obscured by bone metastases.

CLINICAL INTERPRETATION

The appearances are typical of disseminated prostatic carcinoma. Sclerotic bone metastases result in the appearance of increased bone density, whereas the more common lytic bone metastases give an appearance of reduced density in the bone.

In clinical practice, prostate carcinoma is the most common cause of sclerotic lesions. Breast carcinoma usually causes lytic lesions, but may rarely be associated with sclerotic metastases.

Other causes of sclerotic bone lesions (but that will not be widespread as in this case) Include chronic osteomyelitis, primary bone tumours such as osteoma and osteosarcoma, Paget's disease and hyperparathyroidism.

CXR 105

This 60 year old male Presented with Bradyarrhythmia. "sudden breathlessness" Now "peri-arrest"

Q : The most likely cause of this deterioration is:

1. Left ventricular perforation
2. Bowel perforation
3. Tension pneumothorax
4. Left pneumothorax
5. Pericardial effusion

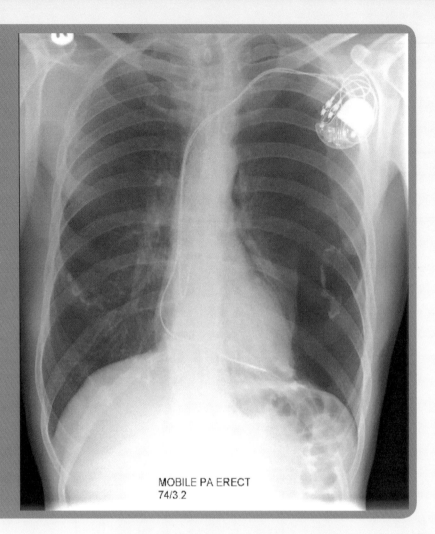

MOBILE PA ERECT
74/3.2

THIS CXR SHOWS

Projection: PA erect. Technically adequate.

Dual chamber pacemaker in situ. Pleural plaques visible over the midzones. There is a large left pneumothorax. Although at present there is minimal mediastinal shift, this clinical presentation is of "tension pneumothorax".

CLINICAL INTERPRETATION

Pneumothorax is a relatively common complication of pacemaker insertion. These may be tolerated well by patients and require no intervention, or require urgent intercostal drainage as in this case.

Tension pneumothorax is characterised by mediastinal shift away from the affected side. Patients are typically severely unwell and require immediate decompression, achieved by inserting a cannulae into the 2nd intercostal space in the mid-clavicular line.

For this reason this is often referred to as the "forbidden chest x-ray"- because if the patient is unwell enough that you suspect a tension pneumothorax you should treat it, not order a chest x-ray!

Answer: 3) Tension Pneumothorax

This 40 year old shoulder has been treated for 4 days for an infected groin sore with flucloxacillin. Now presents with haemoptysis and flu like symptoms. CRP 400mg/l, WCC 0.9 x10⁹/L

CXR 106

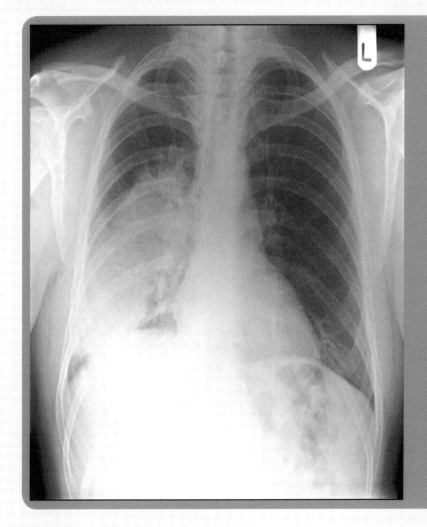

Q: What is the most likely diagnosis?

1. Behcets disease

2. HIV

3. Tuberculosis

4. Community acquired MRSA infection

5. Influenza A pneumonia

THIS CXR SHOWS

Projection: PA, well centred, under penetrated, adequate field of view.

The heart and mediastinum normal. Extensive opacification with air bronchogram in the right mid and lower zone. In addition there is a small area of increased opacification at the left base.

No evidence of pleural effusion or cavitation.

CLINICAL INTERPRETATION

This patient has severe pneumonia due to Panton-Valentine leukocidin positive *staphylococcus aureus*. These are typically community acquired and are often methicillin resistant. Infections with this organism are increasingly recognised. PVL MRSA pneumonia tends to affect young adults, presents with a flu like illness, high fever, haemoptysis and a marked leucopenia (because the PVL toxin destroys white blood cells). There may be a preceding soft tissue infection as in this case, but this is not universal. Mortality is very high[1] and complications include pleural effusion, lung abscess and pulmonary haemorrhage.

[1] Vardakas KZ et al. Incidence, characteristics and outcomes of patients with severe CA-MRSA pneumonia. ERJ. 2009 Jun 18 (epub)

Q : Suggest what treatment this patient has had in the past?

1. Embolisation of arteriovenous malformations

2. Cardiac transplantation surgery

3. Endovascular aortic aneurysm repair

4. Right thoracotomy

5. Thyroidectomy

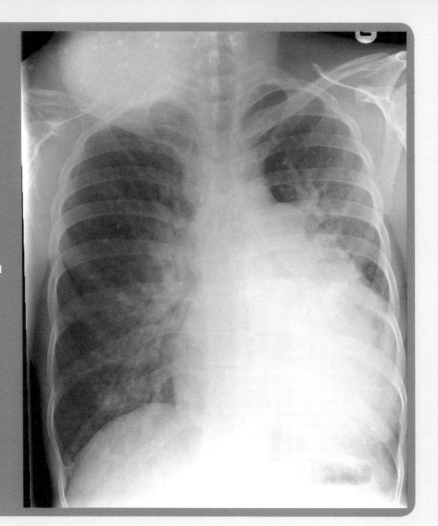

THIS CXR SHOWS

Projection: PA chest x-ray. Technically adequate.

Gross cardiomegaly. Perihilar alveolar opacification bilaterally. Large well-defined abnormality of soft tissue density overlying the right upper zone and extending above the superior aspect of the chest film. There are radio-opaque opacities within the abnormality.

CLINICAL INTERPRETATION

This abnormality is extremely unusual. The patient has a large, complex arteriovenous malformation. The radio-opaque opacities are due to previous attempts at embolisation. The lesion is clearly causing cardiovascular compromise as evidenced by cardiomegaly and peri-hilar opacity that would be consistent with pulmonary oedema.

This is an extreme case, and you would not be expected to immediately reach the diagnosis from the chest film! It is important to have systematic approach and not be distracted by an obvious abnormality.

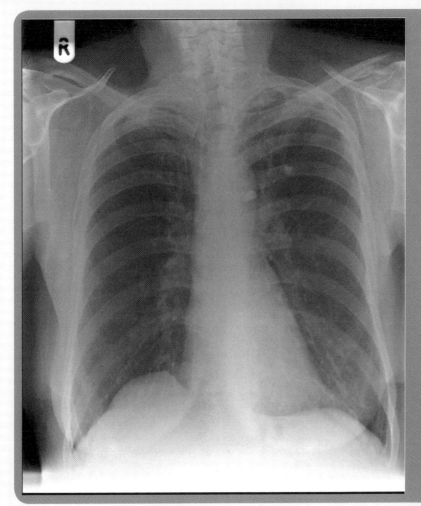

Q : Which of the following is evident on this CXR?

1. Lung carcinoma
2. Carcinoid
3. Cardiomegaly
4. Foreign body aspiration
5. Calcified Granuloma

THIS CXR SHOWS

Projection: PA film. Technically adequate.

Hyperinflated lung fields. Prominent pulmonary vessels. There are calcified granulomas scattered throughout both upper zones.

CLINICAL INTERPRETATION

This lady has had previous TB infection. Calcified granulomas are a common finding in people who have had previous TB infection.

Bacilli are deposited within the terminal airspaces of the lung. Macrophages ingest and transport the bacteria to regional lymph nodes.

Bacilli have 4 potential fates:

1. Elimination by the immune system
2. Multiplying and causing primary TB
3. They may become dormant and cause no clinical disease (latent TB)
4. They may proliferate after a latent period and reactivate (secondary TB). This may occur following 2 and 3.

Q: Immediate treatment should include all except:

1. Oxygen
2. Intravenous opiate
3. Intravenous diuretics
4. Nitrates
5. Thrombolysis

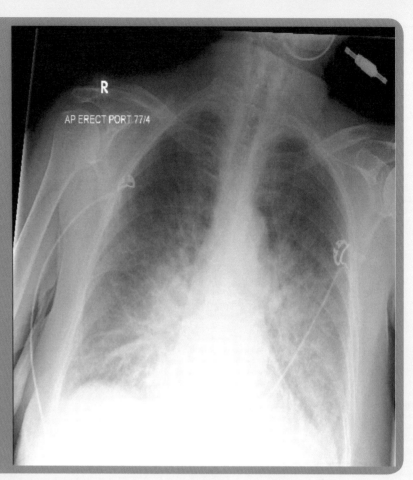

R

AP ERECT PORT 77/4

THIS CXR SHOWS

Projection: PA film, Left costophrenic angle not captured by the film.

There is perihilar "bats wing" shadowing with upper lobe venous diversion.

CLINICAL INTERPRETATION

Although the film quality is poor, this is a typical example of pulmonary oedema. Patients are usually too unwell to pose for a perfect chest film!

The classical features of pulmonary oedema are

- Bilateral alveolar shadowing
- Bilateral pleural effusions
- Cardiomegaly
- Kerly B Lines
- Upper lobe venous diversion

Immediate management should be second nature to all physicians- oxygen, diuretics, nitrates and opiates are the pillars of treatment- followed by treatment of the underlying cause (in this case, acute myocardial infarction).

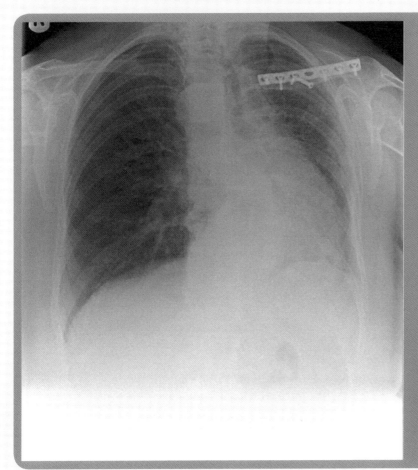

Q: Which of the following would cause tracheal deviation to the left

1. Right pneumonectomy
2. Left pneumothorax
3. Large right pleural effusion
4. RLL collapse
5. Right upper lobe fibrosis

THIS CXR SHOWS

Projection: rotated, adequately inspired and penetrated.

Internal fixation of the left clavicle indicating previous fracture

Mediastinum shifted to the left. Heart apparently enlarged. Right sided aortic arch. Hiatus hernia.

There is medistinal shift to the left indicating decreased volume. There is compensatory enlargement of the right lung. Right lung field clear.

CLINICAL INTERPRETATION

This is an unusual case. The patient has a hypoplastic left lung (congenital). The left lung volume is reduced, leading to mediastinal shift evident on the film. Recognising volume loss is important in interpreting chest x-rays. The mediastinum will usually move towards the affected side. The trachea will deviate towards the side that has lost volume- most commonly in upper lobe collapse. The cardiac shadow will move towards the affected side, usually in lower lobe collapse.

The exceptions are in massive pleural effusions and in tension pneumothorax when the increased pressure in the affected lung will push the mediastinum away from the affected side.

Q : What is the most likely contributing factor to her breathlessness on this CXR?

1. Pulmonary arterial hypertension
2. Pulmonary embolism
3. Pulmonary venous hypertension
4. Arteriovenous malformation
5. Pneumothorax

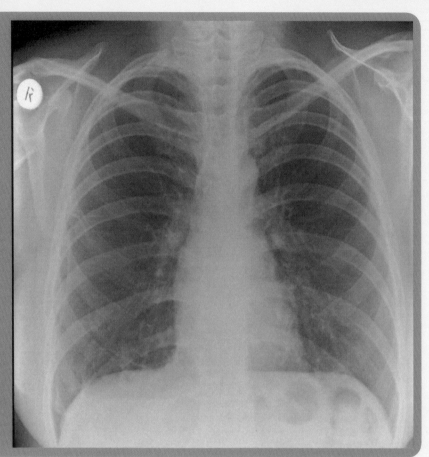

THIS CXR SHOWS

Projection: PA film. Technically adequate.

Hyperinflated lung fields.

There is a small right pneumothorax. The lung edge is most easily visible in the right mid zone.

CLINICAL INTERPRETATION

Neurofibromatosis type I is an autosomal Dominant condition characterised by cutaneous neurofibromas, Café-au-lait spots and Lisch nodules (pigmented spots on the iris). Involvement of the lungs is unusual, Chest wall neurofibromas, kyphoscoliosis and other chest wall deformities are more common.

Bullous lung disease with recurrent pneumothoraces, and interstitial lung disease have been reported[1].

This lady had severe cystic lung disease associated with neurofibromatosis. An important differential diagnosis in young women with cystic lung disease is Lymphangioleiomyomatosis

[1] Eur Respir J 2007; 29:210-214

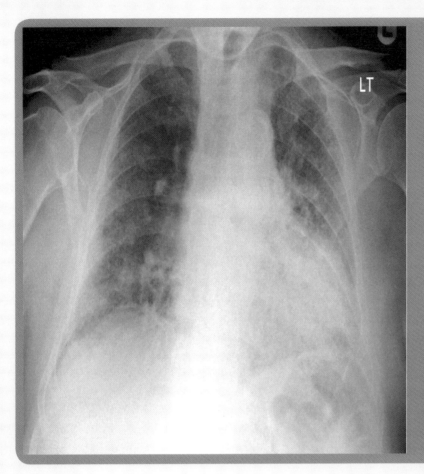

Q : Recognised associations do not include:

1. Nitrofurantoin
2. Asbestos exposure
3. Rheumatoid arthritis
4. Radiotherapy
5. Trimethoprim

THIS CXR SHOWS

Projection: AP erect, rotated. Adequate inspiration and penetration.

Coarse, predominantly peripheral reticular nodular shadowing bilaterally.

CLINICAL INTERPRETATION

This is an example of interstitial lung disease (Idiopathic pulmonary fibrosis).

Diagnosis is made by High Resolution CT scanning.

Recognised underlying causes of interstitial lung disease include:

- Drugs (nitrofurantoin/amiodarone/methotrexate)
- Connective tissue disease (RA)
- Radiation
- Occupation (asbestos, silica)
- Sarcoidosis
- Chronic aspiration

Immunosuppressive treatment is often used. But there is little evidence of benefit. High dose N-acetylcysteine may slow the rate of lung function decline.[1]

Lung transplantation may be considered for a small proportion of patients

[1] N Engl J Med 2005;353:2229-2242

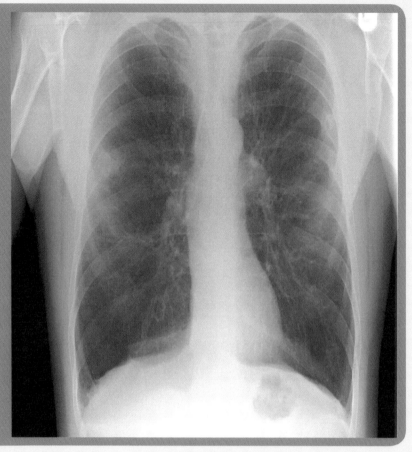

Q : This x-ray shows

1. Hyperinflation
2. RMZ mass lesion
3. Pulmonary hypertension
4. Cystic bronchiectasis
5. Hiatus hernia

THIS CXR SHOWS

Projection: PA film. Technically adequate

Multiple, bilateral rib fractures clear. Features of hyperinflation with generally increased lung markings.

CLINICAL INTERPRETATION

Inflation should be assessed on all chest x-rays. On a correctly inspired film the diaphragm should be seen at the level of the 8th-10th posterior ribs or the right 6th anterior rib. Greater than this is considered hyperinflation.

Other features that suggest hyperinflation
- Flat diaphragms
- Small heart (the heart is not actually small   it just appears that way because the lungs are larger than normal)
- Decreased lung markings in the upper zones. This is a sign of emphysema which often accompanies hyperinflation.

Cannabis abuse is a cause of emphysema and can affect young people quite severely.[1]

Alpha-1-antitrypsin deficiency should be excluded in young patients presenting with emphysema.

[1] Large lung bullae in marijuana smokers Thorax 2000;55:340-342

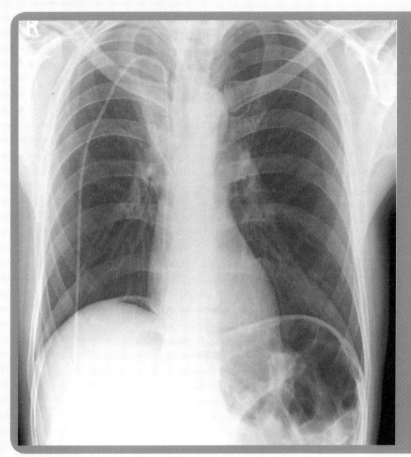

Q: The following is *not* present on this chest x-ray:

1. Pneumoperitoneum
2. Splenic haematoma
3. Jugular venous catheter
4. Elevation of the horizontal fissure
5. Tracheal deviation to the right

THIS CXR SHOWS

Projection: PA film. Technically adequate

Central venous cannulae in situ with tip in right atrium.

Bilateral air beneath the diaphragm

Triangular opacity projected medially in the right upper zone. Tracheal deviation to right.

CLINICAL INTERPRETATION

The patient has clearly had abdominal surgery as suggested by the air under the diaphragms. If the introduction did not say that this patient is post-op, you would suspect a perforated abdominal viscus.

Junior doctors are often asked to check the position of central venous lines. These should lie in the lower superior vena cava at the level of the carina, not in the right atrium.

Right upper lobe collapse may occur post-operatively due to mucous plugging. It should be recognised on the chest x-ray as a triangular opacity in the right upper zone.

The borders of the triangle are formed by the horizontal fissure which moves upwards and the border of the superior mediastinum.

RUL collapse will usually be accompanied by movement of the trachea towards the affected side.

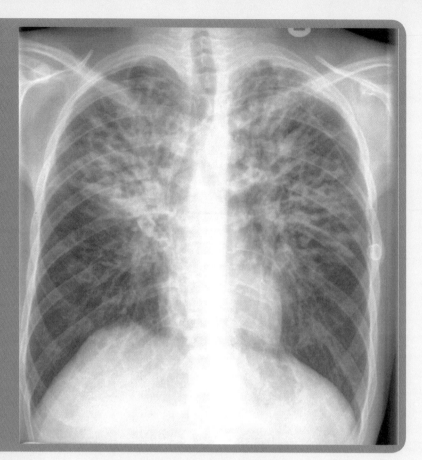

Q: Sputum culture is likely to yield which organism

1. *Pseudomonas aeruginosa*
2. *Moraxella catarhalis*
3. *Haemophilus influenzae*
4. *Streptococcus pneumoniae*
5. *Mycobacterium avium complex*

THIS CXR SHOWS

Projection: PA film. Technically adequate

Left subcutaneous venous access port ("portacath")

Gross changes of bronchiectasis with bronchial wall thickening and dilatation, scarring and cystic change particularly in the perihilar regions bilaterally.

CLINICAL INTERPRETATION

Cystic fibrosis lung disease is characterised by severe bronchiectasis. Bronchiectasis is dilation of the bronchi. This dilation prevents effective clearance of mucous, impairing innate pulmonary defences and leading to colonisation of the normally sterile respiratory tract with bacteria.

In the UK, patients with cystic fibrosis are usually managed by a multi-disciplinary team in specialist units. However, patients may be admitted to general medical units with other problems, or to district general hospitals if they live far from a specialist unit. It is important, therefore, to recognise the x-ray changes of cystic fibrosis. Old x-rays are particularly useful as patients may feel very well with gross bronchiectatic changes on the chest x-ray.

Clinically, changes in lung function and patient reported symptoms and quality of life are more useful than x-ray severity.

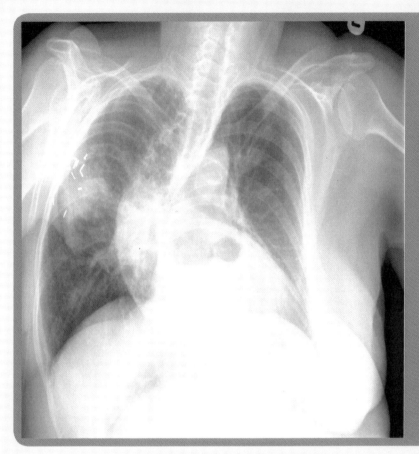

Q: Which of the following features is not present on this chest x-ray:

1. RMZ consolidation
2. Previous breast surgery
3. Hiatus hernia
4. Tracheal deviation
5. Scoliosis

THIS CXR SHOWS

Projection: PA film. Severe scoliosis. Adequate penetration.

Right axillary surgical clips.

Hiatus hernia.

Marked chest wall deformity.

Alveolar based shadowing particularly in the RLZ.

Some streaky opacification in the medial LUZ.

Patchy opacification overlying the RMZ.

CLINICAL INTERPRETATION

This lady has had previous lumpectomy for breast carcinoma with axillary clearance. She did not have alveolar hypoventilation on arterial blood gases despite the gross chest wall deformity.

CT chest was requested to look for other explanations such as lymphangitis, lung metastases and radiation pneumonitis.

No obvious explanation was found. Recurrent aspiration is a possible diagnosis.

Q : Other features associated with this syndrome include:

1. Increased 24 hour urinary calcium excretion

2. Positive rheumatoid factor

3. Reduced diffusion capacity on pulmonary function testing

4. Red cell casts on urine microscopy

5. Elevated CA-125

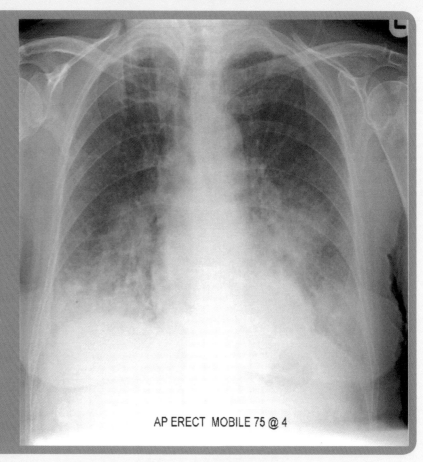

AP ERECT MOBILE 75 @ 4

THIS CXR SHOWS

Projection: AP erect

Pulmonary: Alveolar shadowing affecting both mid to lower zones.

CLINICAL INTERPRETATION

Pulmonary-renal syndromes include Wegener's granulomatosis and anti-glomerular basement membrane syndrome (Goodpastures syndrome).

They present with haemoptysis and renal failure.

There is often upper respiratory tract symptoms

In association with Wegener's- rhinitis is often the first symptom.

cANCA positivity can aid the diagnosis but is not specific. The chest x-ray appearances are variable and may include nodules, cavities or infiltrates as in this case. Bilateral infiltrates may be the result of pulmonary haemorrhage.

The American College of Rheumatology diagnostic Criteria[1] requires 2/4 of

- Haematuria or red cell casts on urine microscopy
- Abnormal chest x-ray
- Nasal or oral inflammation
- A positive biopsy for granulomatous inflammation

[1] Arthritis Rheum. 1990 Aug;33(8):1101-7.

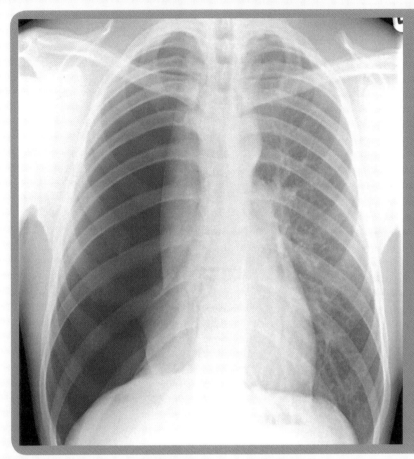

Q : The most appropriate management would be:

1. Observation

2. Therapeutic pleural aspiration

3. Intercostal drainage

4. Thoracoscopic pleurectomy

5. Thoracotomy with pleurectomy

THIS CXR SHOWS

Projection: PA film. Technically adequate.

Complete right pneumothorax. No evidence of mediastinal shift

CLINICAL INTERPRETATION

This is primary pneumothorax- pneumothorax in a patient without a history of chronic lung disease. Patients are typically tall and thin. Cigarette smoking is a predisposing factor.

Current British Thoracic society guidelines recommend that symptomatic patients (as in this case) should initially receive needle aspiration and if necessary a second aspiration procedure before insertion of an intercostal drain. In practice many of these patients are managed with intercostal drainage.

Asymptomatic patients with a rim of air <2cm may be managed without further treatment with the expectation that the pneumothorax will resolve spontaneously.

★ ★

Answer: 2) Therapeutic pleural aspiration

Q : The following are causes of elevated hemidiaphragm, except:

1. Subphrenic abscess
2. Pulmonary embolism
3. Phrenic nerve palsy
4. Aortic aneurysm
5. Ectopic pregnancy

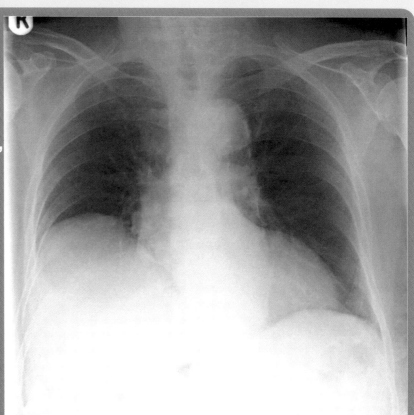

THIS CXR SHOWS

Projection: PA film. Technically adequate.

Unfolded aorta with calcification.

Raised right hemidiaphragm.

Clear lung fields

CLINICAL INTERPRETATION

The x-ray shows elevation of the right hemi-diaphragm. This may be asymptomatic and an incidental finding or may indicate significant pathology.

Because the right hemi-diaphragm is normally higher than the left, subtle elevation may be easily missed. A difference in height between the right and left hemidiaphragms of >3cm usually indicates significant pathology.

Causes of elevation of the right hemidiaphragm include:

- Phrenic nerve palsy
- Malignancy
- Cervical spinal disease
- Aortic Aneurysm
- Congenital
- Pulmonary Disease
- Volume loss (e.g. pulmonary infarct/lobectomy)
- Subdiaphragmatic disease
- Subphrenic abscess
- Peritonitis
- Distension of colon or stomach

Answer: 5) Ectopic pregnancy

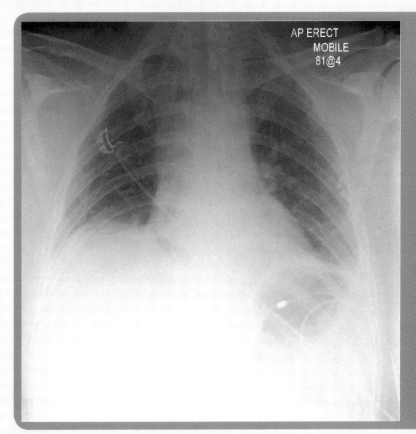

Q: Gall stones are visible on Plain x-ray in....

1. 1%
2. 10%
3. 20%
4. 50%
5. 70%

THIS CXR SHOWS

Projection: AP erect film. Under-inspired

Oxygen tubing and ECG electrodes visible.

There is left lower zone shadowing suggesting a possible effusion but the film is suboptimal to assess for this.

There is a nasogastric tube coiled in the stomach. No gallstones are visible.

CLINICAL INTERPRETATION

This lady had gallstone pancreatitis. Only around 10% of gallstones are calcified enough to be visible on x-ray as the majority are composed of cholesterol which is radio-opaque.

Standard conservative management consists of intravenous hydration, nil by mouth and nasogastric tube drainage.

Pancreatitis may be associated with pleural effusion. This is an exudate and pleural fluid amylase levels may be detected in high concentrations.

Q : What long term treatment does this lady require?

1. Indwelling pleural drain
2. Corticosteroids
3. Pulsed cyclophosphamide
4. Penicillin
5. Low dose macrolide

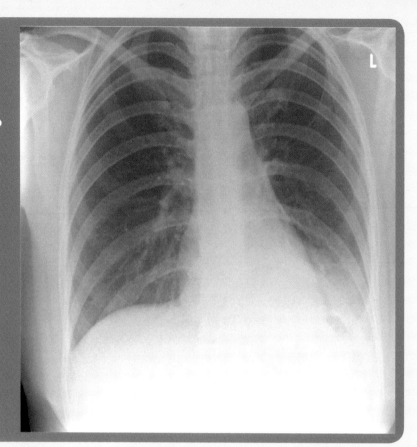

THIS CXR SHOWS

Projection: PA film, technically adequate

There is homogenous opacification of the left hemi-diaphragm with blunting of the costophrenic angle consistent with a pleural effusion.

CLINICAL INTERPRETATION

This lady has a post-operative left pleural effusion. Diagnostic pleural aspiration should be performed.

In this case the lady had developed a post operative pneumonia with parapneumonic effusion.

Splenectomy carries a long term risk of infections from capsulated organisms such as *Streptococcus pneumoniae* and *Haemophilus Influenzae*. Antibiotic prophylaxis with penicillin is recommended.

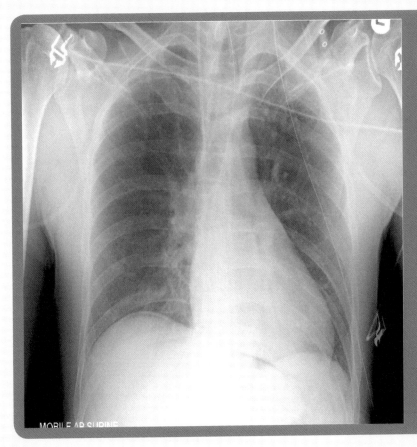

Q: The following are features present on this CXR except:

1. Elevated right hemidiaphragm

2. Internal jugular venous line

3. Pneumoperitoneum

4. Oxygen tubing

5. Increased cardiothoracic ratio

THIS CXR SHOWS

Projection: AP erect film, rotated.

ECG electrodes and oxygen tubing visible. There is a right internal jugular venous line with the tip in the superior vena cava.

There is a thin rim of air beneath the right hemi-diaphragm.

There is alveolar opacification within the left upper zone.

CLINICAL INTERPRETATION

There are a large number of abnormalities on this chest film. It is important to take a systematic approach like the method described in this book to avoid being distracted by an obvious abnormality, and therefore missing a more subtle one (such as air under the diaphragm).

The presenting symptom is abdominal pain and there is air under the diaphragm. A perforated viscus is the most likely diagnosis. In addition there is patchy opacification in the LUZ in this case, it was due to infection.

Evidence of pneumoperitoneum can be seen on plain films in only 75% of cases of perforated viscus and CT abdomen is required to exclude this if clinically suspected.

Q: Which of the following is an indication for large bore drain insertion?

1. Primary pneumothorax

2. Secondary pneumothorax

3. Exudate pleural effusion

4. Haemothorax

5. Hepatic hydrothorax

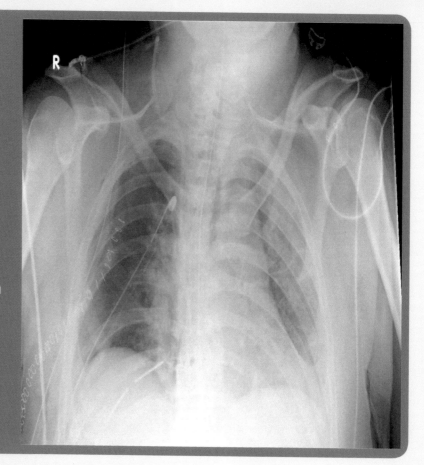

THIS CXR SHOWS

Projection: AP erect film

ECG electrodes visible.

There are surgical clips and ribs resected over the right hemithorax from a right thoracotomy. Central venous catheter with the tip at the level of the carina.

There are 2 large bore chest drains inserted within the right pleural space.

CLINICAL INTERPRETATION

As with the previous case, chest x-rays with multiple abnormalities can feel overwhelming if you have not had much experience of patients Who have undergone major surgery and/or require intensive care.

A systematic approach is the key to avoid being distracted by the obvious abnormalities and therefore missing the more subtle ones.

The patient has 2 large bore chest drains in situ following this surgery. The fenestrations on the Intercostal drains can be clearly seen in the Image.

There has been a recent decline in the use of large bore chest drains. BTS guidelines now recommend 12F chest drains, inserted using the seldinger technique for the majority of indications including initial management of pneumothorax and pleural effusion.

Empyema and haemothorax (such as may occur post operatively) are important exceptions and may require large bore drain insertion.

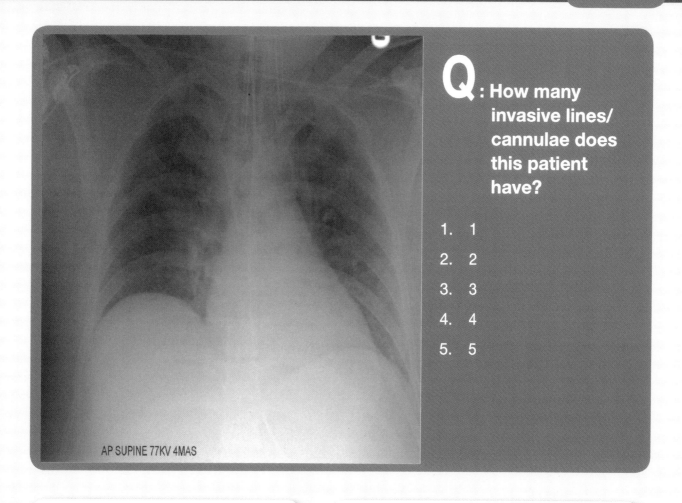

AP SUPINE 77KV 4MAS

Q: How many invasive lines/ cannulae does this patient have?

1. 1
2. 2
3. 3
4. 4
5. 5

THIS CXR SHOWS

Projection: AP supine film. Over penetrated

ECG electrodes and oxygen tubing visible. Central venous line in-situ. endotracheal tube and nasogastric tube also present.

CLINICAL INTERPRETATION

This is the typical appearance of a patient ventilated on the intensive care unit. Various lines are required for intensive monitoring and are evident on the chest x-ray. All doctors should be familiar with these lines as they will often be asked to check their position. The CVP line can be seen clearly with the tip in the superior vena cava.

The endotracheal tube is visible following the line of the trachea. The nasogastric tube disappears off the bottom of the chest x-ray and so its precise location is uncertain.

Q: What is the cause of the "white out"?

1. Iatrogenic
2. Malignant effusion
3. Tension pneumothorax
4. Pneumonectomy
5. Obstructed left main bronchus

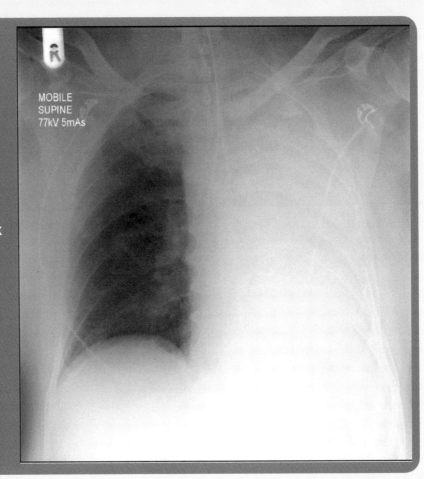

MOBILE
SUPINE
77kV 5mAs

THIS CXR SHOWS

Projection: AP supine film

There is consolidation in the right upper lobe.

There is complete opacification over the left hemithorax with mediastinal shift to the left in keeping with collapse.

There is an ET tube within the right main bronchus.

CLINICAL INTERPRETATION

This gentleman has been intubated following his cardiac arrest. Unfortunately the ET tube has been misplaced into the right main bronchus. As a result the left lung is not being ventilated. The problem can be easily corrected by pulling the endotracheal tube back into the trachea. Compare the position of the endotracheal tube in this film with the previous film.

In a "white out", look immediately for mediastinal shift. Shift usually indicates collapse (with the mediastinum moving towards the collapse). Occasionally, a massive pleural effusion will cause the mediastinum to shift away from the effusion.

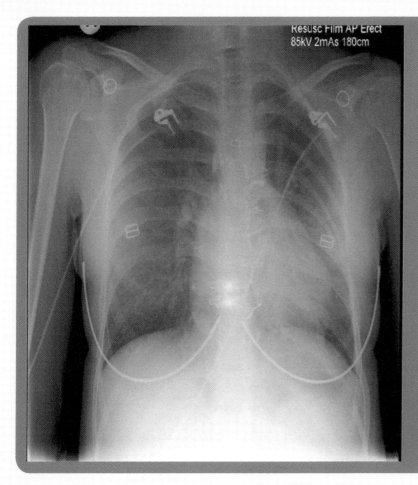

Resusc Film AP Erect
85kV 2mAs 180cm

Q: Which structure is **not** visible on this chest x-ray?

1. Left ventricle
2. Right ventricle
3. Left atrium
4. Right atrium
5. Pulmonary artery

THIS CXR SHOWS

Projection: AP erect film.

Bra wiring and clips visible. ECG electrodes visible. Sternotomy wires indicate previous cardiac surgery.

There is a radiolucent object in the mediastinum indicating a pulmonary artery stent. There are multiple coils from embolisation of collateral blood vessels.

CLINICAL INTERPRETATION

This young lady was born with hypoplastic right heart syndrome. Many patients have chest x-rays like this showing evidence of childhood surgery and subsequent medical procedures.

The mediastinal contours on the chest x-ray give information about the heart and related structures. Remember that on a normal PA film, the right ventricle is not visible as it lies anteriorly. The right heart border is made by right atrium. The left heart border is made up of the left atrium and left ventricle. The left side of the heart accounts for at least 2/3 of the cardiac shadow visible on the PA chest x-ray.

The overall cardiac size should make no more than half of the thoracic cavity.

Q: **You suspect asbestosis. Which of the following investigations would you like to perform?**

1. Transbronchial lung biopsy

2. Bronchoalveolar lavage (BAL)

3. High resolution CT chest (HRCT)

4. Spirometry

5. Pleural biopsy

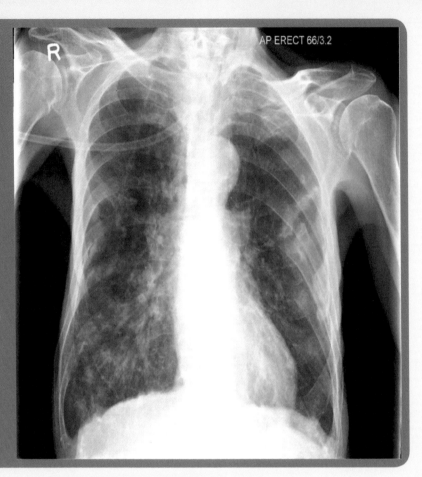

AP ERECT 66/3.2

THIS CXR SHOWS

Projection: AP erect film. Oxygen tubing visible

There is hyperinflation of the lung fields. There are multiple pleural plaques, most evident in the left mid-zone peripherally.

There is no obvious associated fibrosis.

CLINICAL INTERPRETATION

Asbestos exposure is a major cause of respiratory mortality and morbidity. The epidemic of asbestosis has probably reached its peak but mesothelioma probably hasn't.

Commonly patients give a history of working in trades such as ship-building, construction, heating and insulation (and roofing), or factory work.

Disorders associated with asbestos exposure include

- Pleural plaques
- Asbestos related diffuse pleural thickening
- Benign asbestosis related pleural effusions
- Asbestosis (pulmonary fibrosis)
- Bronchial Carcinoma
- Mesothelioma

Pleural plaques do not cause respiratory symptoms but can cause significant worry and distress to patients

Answer: High resolution CT chest (HRCT)

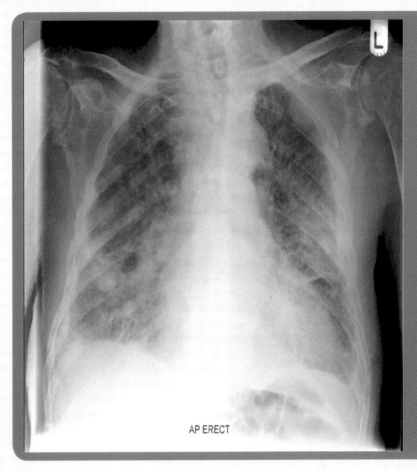

AP ERECT

Q: Which 2 diagnoses explain this x-ray appearance?

1. Prostate carcinoma and left pneumonia

2. Breast carcinoma with pleural metastases

3. Prostate carcinoma with lung metastases

4. Hepatocellular carcinoma and trans-diaphragmatic invasion

5. Prostate carcinoma and acute myocardial infarction

THIS CXR SHOWS

Projection: AP erect film.

Oxygen mask in situ.

Sclerotic bone metastases visible with complete destruction of the left first rib

AP film limits assessment, however heart appears enlarged.

There is perihilar alveolar shadowing most obvious on the left but also present on the right.

CLINICAL INTERPRETATION

The chest x-ray shows pulmonary oedema in a patient with disseminated prostate carcinoma. The pulmonary oedema followed an acute myocardial infarction.

Also see x-ray 104 for a discussion of bone metastases.

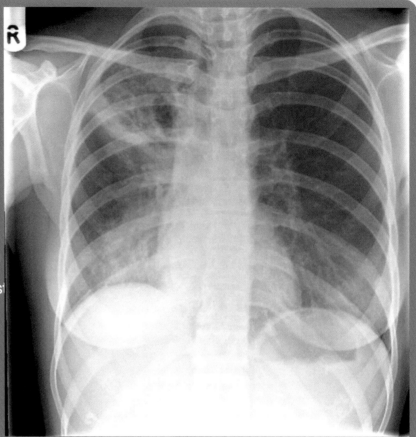

Q: The following parameters indicate severe pneumonia except?

1. Urea 8.1mmol/l
2. Respiratory 30/min
3. Blood pressure 108/60
4. Abbreviated mental test score 7/10
5. C-reactive protein 320mg/l

THIS CXR SHOWS

Projection: PA film. Technically adequate

Obliteration of the right heart border.

There is consolidation with air-bronchograms in the right upper, middle and lower zones.

CLINICAL INTERPRETATION

The chest x-ray shows multilobar pneumonia.
The most likely cause is bacterial community acquired pneumonia.
The causative organism cannot be reliably determined based on either clinical presentation or chest x-ray appearances.
The British Thoracic Society recommend a severity guided approach to management with All patients being assessed using the CURB65 score on hospital admission. This is calculated as

Confusion – new onset

Urea – Raised > 7mmol/l

Respiratory rate - Raised ≥ 30/minute

Blood pressure (systolic <90 mmHg *and*/or diastolic ≤60 mmHg)

Age ≥ **65** years

A score of ≥3 indicates severe pneumonia

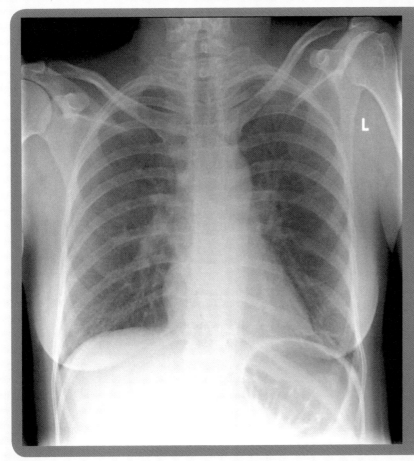

Q : Koplik spots indicate a diagnosis of:

1. Histoplasmosis

2. HIV seroconversion illness

3. Pregnancy

4. Measles

5. Epstein Barr virus infection

THIS CXR SHOWS

Projection: PA film. Technically adequate

Minor atelectasis at the left base. No other abnormality

CLINICAL INTERPRETATION

This lady has measles. The chest x-ray is essentially normal. Measles rates have increased in recent years in the UK. This is believed to be due to a decrease in the uptake of the combined measles, mumps and rubella vaccination (MMR) which effectively prevents the disease.

Controversial claims linking the vaccination to autism, which have subsequently been discredited, have been blamed for the poor uptake. In 2007, 85% of children were vaccinated, well below the 95% required to produce "Herd Immunity" effectively eradicating the potential for measles outbreaks.

Measles pneumonitis is extremely rare but serious complication of the disease. There is no evidence of this in the present case.

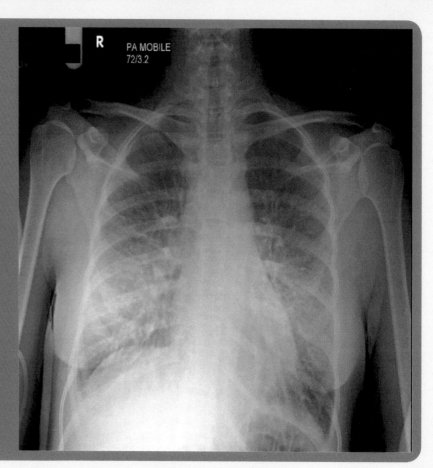

Q : The chest x-ray shows

1. Bilateral pneumonia
2. Bilateral empyema
3. Right pulmonary embolism
4. Flash pulmonary oedema
5. LLL collapse

THIS CXR SHOWS

Projection: PA film. Technically adequate

Bilateral lower zone/perihilar alveolar shadowing consistent with acute pneumonia.

Left basal atelectasis still present.

CLINICAL INTERPRETATION

Measles pneumonitis is a serious complication with a high mortality rate. In adults, patients are usually extremely hypoxic and other atypical features including thrombocytopenia, hepatitis, myositis and hypocalcaemia have been reported.[1]

Intravenous Ribavirin has been used effectively to treat the disease. Patients often require mechanical ventilation and supportive treatment.

Cases such as these should inform the public debate about a preventable disease.

[1] Severe Measles Pneumonitis in Adults: Evaluation Of clinical characteristics and therapy with IV ribavirin Clin Infect Dis 1994;19(3):454-62.

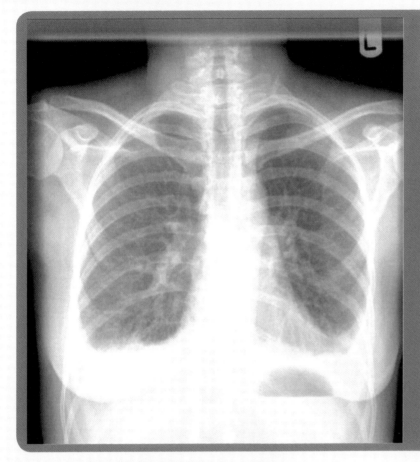

Q: A pleural tap is performed- which of the following indicate an exudate:

1. Pleural Protein 29g/L
2. Pleural Protein 37g/L
3. Serum albumin 45g/L
4. LDH 231iu/L
5. Pleural pH 7.25

THIS CXR SHOWS

Projection: PA film. Technically adequate

Bilateral pleural effusions

CLINICAL INTERPRETATION

This unusual case is now resolving. The pneumonitis is gone and she is left with bilateral reactive pleural effusions.

Pleural effusions are common, affecting 25-50% of patients with pneumonia. Parapneumonic effusions are usually exudates. These can be recognised by Lights Criteria[1] as

- Pleural fluid protein > 0.5x serum protein
- Pleural fluid LDH > 0.6x serum LDH
- Pleural fluid LDH > 2/3 the upper limit of normal

Lights criteria has a higher sensitivity than pleural protein alone.

[1] Parapneumonic Effusions Am J Med. 1980;69(4):507-12.

Q: Which of the following features does **not** indicate a poor prognosis?

1. Bilateral shadowing
2. Oxygen saturation 94%
3. Pleural effusion
4. Confusion
5. Age of 86 years

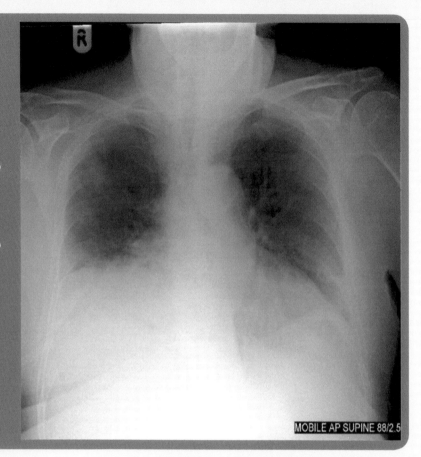

MOBILE AP SUPINE 88/2.5

THIS CXR SHOWS

Projection: AP film. Under-inspired. Over penetrated.

Bilateral dense lower zone alveolar shadowing. Upper lobe venous diversion.

CLINICAL INTERPRETATION

Bilateral pneumonia carries a worse prognosis. Other radiological features associated with increased mortality are multilobar shadowing and pleural effusions.[1]

Presenting symptoms are often less clear cut in elderly patients. Patients aged > 65 years are more likely to present with acute confusion, unexplained pyrexia or collapse, and are less likely to give the classical symptoms of cough, sputum production and breathlessness.

The causative organism may be different in elderly patients. Patients aged >65 years are more likely to have pneumonia caused by *haemophilus influenzae, moraxella catarhalis* and gram negative organisms. *Mycoplasma pneumoniae, legionella pneumophilia* and respiratory viruses are more common in younger patients in the UK.[2]

[1] A prediction rule to identify low-risk patients with community-acquired pneumonia. *N Engl J Med* 1997;336:243-250

[2] British Thoracic Society Guidelines for the management of community Acquired pneumonia in Adults. Update 2009.

Answer: 2) Oxygen saturation 94%

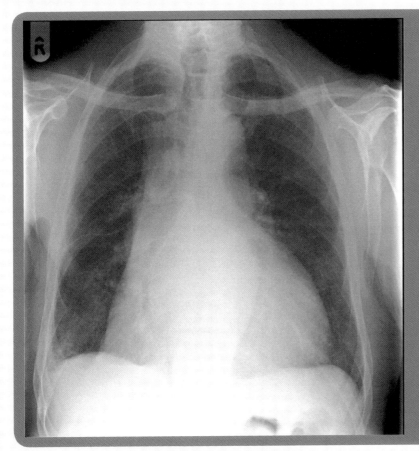

Q: The following are recognised causes of cardiomegaly except:

1. Pericardial effusion

2. Hypertension

3. Glycogen storage disease

4. Hypertrophic Obstructive Cardiomyopathy (HOCM)

5. *Pneumocystis Jerovici pneumonia*

THIS CXR SHOWS

Projection: PA, right rotation, under penetrated, adequate field of view.

There is gross cardiomegaly and a hiatus hernia visible behind the heart border. There is also some hazy opacification at the right costophrenic angle possibly due to pleural thickening.

CLINICAL INTERPRETATION

Cardiomegaly is usually present if the maximum width of the cardiac silhouette is more than 50% of the maximum internal diameter of the rib cage. Cardiomegaly alone rarely correlates with abnormal findings on echocardiography. However, in the context of clinical features suggestive of cardiac disease and abnormal ECG findings, more than 60% of patients will have an abnormal Echocardiography study.[1]

[1] European Journal of Echocardiography 2007 8(3):s33

Q : Which lobe of the lung is involved?

1. RUL
2. RUL anterior segment
3. RML superior segment
4. RML inferior segment
5. RLL apical segment

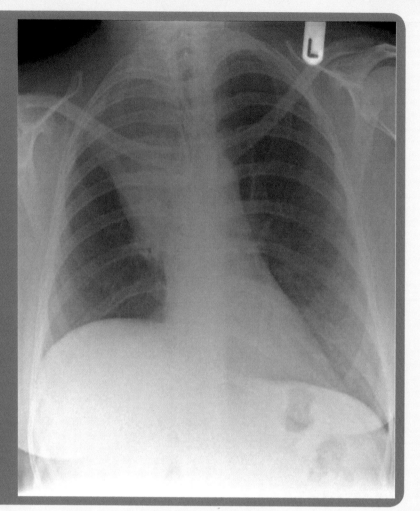

THIS CXR SHOWS

Projection: PA film

There is opacification of the right upper zone. The horizontal fissure is pulled up indicating right upper lobe collapse. The right hilum is enlarged.

CLINICAL INTERPRETATION

Malignancy is the most common cause of lobar collapse presenting to outpatient clinics. Right upper lobe collapse presents as a triangular opacity in the upper lung field. There is elevation of the horizontal fissure and deviation of the trachea to the affected side. Where the lesion is due to a right hilar mass there is often a bulge (the mass) at the base of the triangle.

This is known as Golden's "S" sign

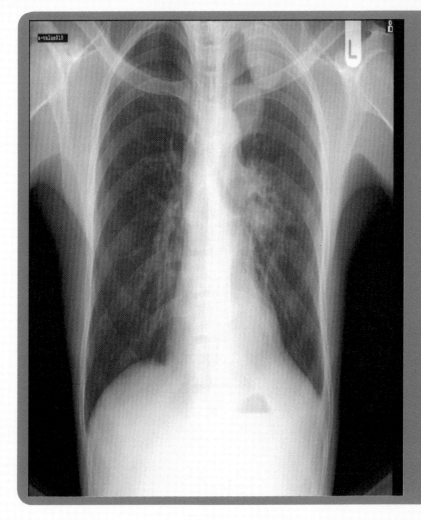

Q : What is the likely diagnosis?

1. Mycobacterium Leprae

2. Syphilis

3. Sarcoidosis

4. Mycobacterium avium intracellulare

5. Mycobacterium tuberculosis

THIS CXR SHOWS

Projection: PA film. Technically adequate

There is a soft tissue mass in the left upper zone overlying the 1st and 2nd posterior ribs and the left clavicle. complete loss of the left hemidiaphragm and blunting of the costophrenic angle.

There is enlargement of the left hilum with dilated bronchi suggesting bronchiectasis here.

CLINICAL INTERPRETATION

This is a complex case with multiple abnormalities again emphasising the important of a systematic approach. The soft tissue mass in the left upper zone is clearly separate from the lung (which can be seen underneath) and was a further abscess.

The loss of the left hemidiaphragm and left lower zone volume loss suggests left lower lobe collapse. Hilar enlargement causing lower lobe collapse is well recognised in tuberculosis which seems a likely unifying diagnosis in this case.

★ ★

Answer: 5) Mycobacterium Tuberculosis

Q : The following features are visible on this chest x-ray except:

1. Intercostal drain
2. Right pleural effusion
3. Left pleural effusion
4. Nodules
5. Thoracic vertebrae

AP ERECT MOBILE 86/22

THIS CXR SHOWS

Projection: AP film. Underpenetrated, underinspired.

The patient is obese. there are multiple rounded soft tissue opacities in both lung fields consistent with pulmonary metastases.

Bilateral pleural effusions.

CLINICAL INTERPRETATION

This is a case of metastatic breast carcinoma. The film is of very poor quality and illustrates some of the difficulties in interpreting chest films in the emergency department. Often it is better to request a repeat film rather than attempt to interpret a sub-optimal film.

To illustrate the point, this lady actually has a left intercostal chest drain in situ, but this is not visible on the current film due to underpenetration and the patient's body habitus.

Answer: 1) Intercostal drain

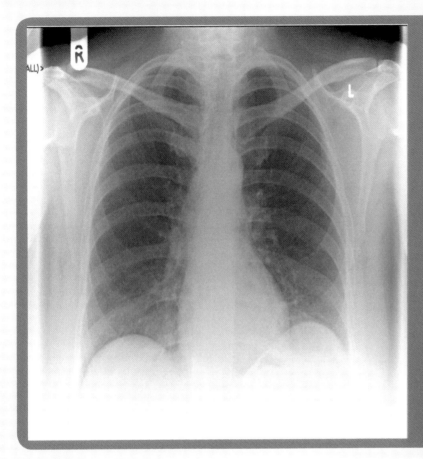

Q: This chest x-ray shows

1. RUL consolidation
2. RLL consolidation
3. LUL cavitation
4. Elevated right hemidiaphragm
5. None of the above

THIS CXR SHOWS

Projection: PA film, technically adequate.

Minor atelectasis at the left base. Otherwise normal.

CLINICAL INTERPRETATION

An essentially normal chest x-ray in a patient with night sweats. Among the common causes for night sweats with a normal CXR include:

- Menopause/perimenopause
- Viral infections
- Abscesses
- Hyperthyroidism
- Lymphoproliferative disorders
- HIV
- Non-pulmonary tuberculosis
- Alcoholism
- Chronic infections (e.g. Brucellosis, Malaria)
- Active Sarcoid

Chest x-ray is not 100% sensitive for detection of bronchial tumours or tuberculosis and in patients with a high risk clinical history (as in this case of a smoker with night sweats) more sensitive imaging with CT is indicated.

The patient was ultimately diagnosed with lymphoma.

Q: The following are more common in pregnancy except:

1. Exacerbation of asthma
2. Pulmonary embolism
3. Aminotic fluid embolism
4. Pneumonia
5. Lymphangioleiomyomatosis

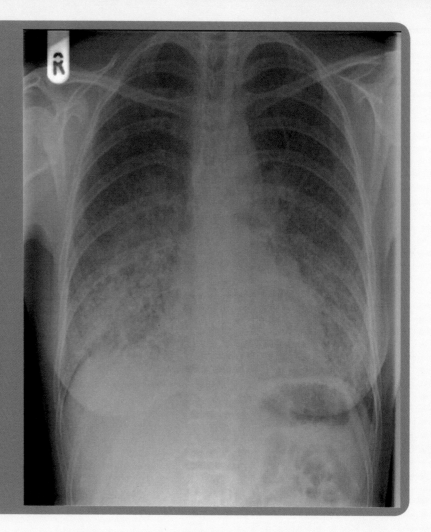

THIS CXR SHOWS

Projection: PA film, technically adequate.

There is a bilateral nodular interstitial infiltrate primarily affecting the lower zones but extending into the upper zones.

CLINICAL INTERPRETATION

Hypoxaemia in a pregnant patient raises diagnostic difficulties. There is reluctance to perform chest x-ray in pregnancy due to a theoretical risk of increasing developmental abnormalities in the foetus. However, the radiation dose associated with plain chest x-ray is equivalent to 3 days of natural background radiation in the UK.

In a patient who is acutely unwell, the risk of not obtaining an accurate diagnosis by CXR outweighs the risk to the foetus.

Asthma and pulmonary embolism are common in pregnancy and are often associated with a normal chest x-ray. Pneumonia, pulmonary oedema and more sinister, rare diagnoses such as disseminated neoplasia (as in this unfortunate case) are thankfully rare.[1]

[1] Respiratory Complications of Pregnancy. Obstet Gynecol Surv. 2002 ;57(1):39-46.

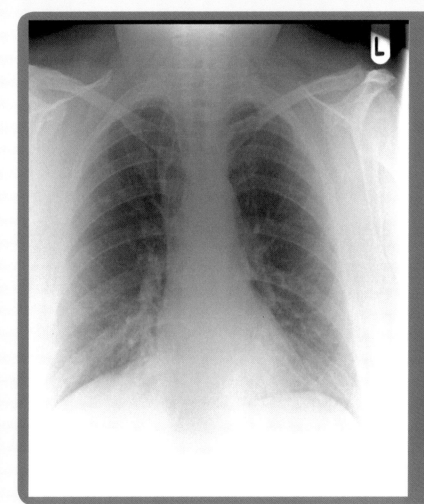

Q: What is the next appropriate intervention?

1. Bronchoscopy

2. CT chest staging

3. Trans-carinal lymph node biopsy

4. Smoking cessation

5. Repeat CXR in 3 months

THIS CXR SHOWS

Projection: PA film, technically adequate.

There is an azygos lobe visible in the right upper zone.

CLINICAL INTERPRETATION

The azygos lobe is a normal variant, present in 0.1–8% of the population which develops when the apex of the right lung encounters the arch of the azygos vein during embryological development.

The azygos lobe is not associated with any pathology and no further investigations or treatment are required.

Q: Arterial blood analysis was abnormal. Which of the following acid-base disturbance is most likely?

1. Compensated type 2 respiratory failure

2. Decompensated type 2 respiratory failure

3. Type 1 respiratory failure

4. Compensated metabolic acidosis

5. Decompensated metabolic acidaemia

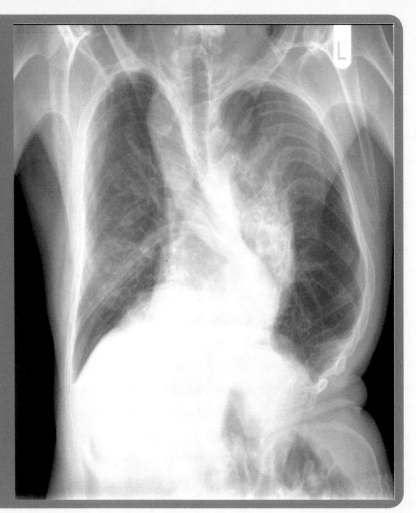

THIS CXR SHOWS

Projection: PA, well centred, adequate penetration, adequate field of view.

Marked kyphoscoliosis of the thoracic spine concave to the left upper lung field and resulting in narrowing of multiple rib spaces.

CLINICAL INTERPRETATION

Kyphoscoliosis describes an abnormal curvature of the spine in both a coronal and saggital plane. It is a combination of kyphosis and scoliosis.

Braces and other orthopaedic interventions at young age may help moderate deformities. Long term sequelae of chest wall deformity is chest wall restriction leading to alveolar hypoventilation and hypercapnia which is detected on arterial blood gas sampling. The respiratory acidosis is compensated by retaining bicarbonate to maintain a normal pH. Symptomatic patients often benefit from non-invasive ventilation.

Answer: 1) Compensated type 2 respiratory failure

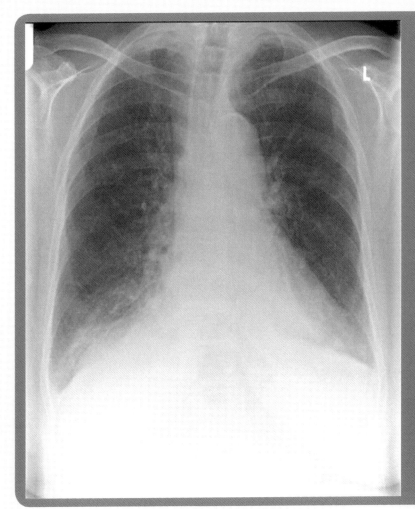

Q : Which of the following would suggest Legionnaires disease?

1. Erythema Multiforme
2. Exposure to birds
3. Erythema nodosum
4. Hyponatraemia
5. Koplik spots

THIS CXR SHOWS

Projection: PA film, technically adequate.

Aortic unfolding and calcification of the arch.

Alveolar shadowing in the right lower zone with loss of the hemidiaphragm suggesting right lower lobe pneumonia.

CLINICAL INTERPRETATION

This lady has community acquired pneumonia with recent foreign travel.

Atypical coverage is essential including *mycoplasma* and *Legionella*. The latter is common in Southern Europe. Antibiotic therapy must also take account of the fact that up to 60% of pneumococci in Southern Europe are penicillin resistant (<10% in the UK). Contrary to what some have held to be true in the past, it is now recognised that there is no uniform presentation or radiographic appearance that allows the atypical pneumonias to be recognised on clinical grounds.

Diagnosis is based on serology testing, urinary antigen testing or more recently the use of PCR based tests from throat swabs.

Q: This chest x-ray shows:

1. Tracheal deviation to the right
2. Left ureteric stone
3. Pulmonary nodule
4. Elevated right hemidiaphragm
5. None of the above

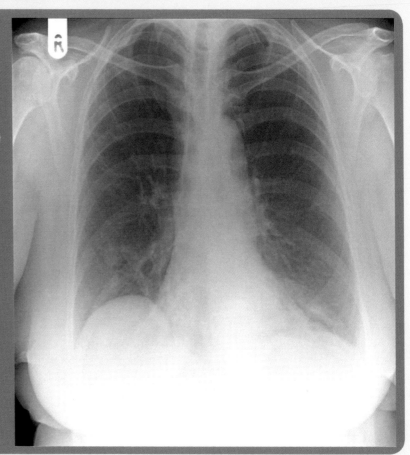

THIS CXR SHOWS

Projection: PA film, technically adequate.

Ill defined opacity approx

2cm in diameter in the right lower zone. Left basal atelectasis. General

paucity of lung markings in the upper zones suggesting emphysema.

CLINICAL INTERPRETATION

Pulmonary nodules are common and do not always represent malignancy. Comparison with previous films is essential. A nodule that is new, or has increased or size is an indicator of likely malignant disease.

CT scanning is mandatory for any patient with a suspicion of malignancy.

Small peripheral lung nodules are rarely amenable to bronchoscopic biopsy and so CT guided lung biopsy is the investigation of choice to confirm the suspicion of lung carcinoma and to determine the histological type. This is crucial to further management.

Answer: 3) Pulmonary nodule ★ ★

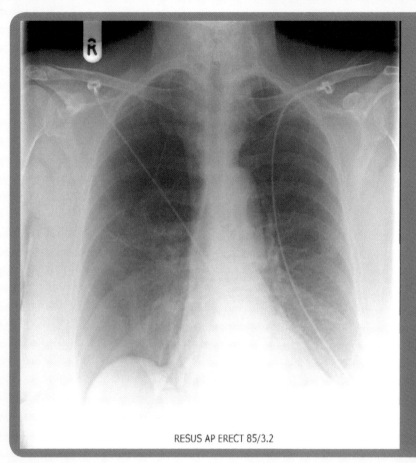

RESUS AP ERECT 85/3.2

Q: Common complications of CT guided lung biopsy Include the following **except:**

1. Pneumonia
2. Pulmonary haemorrhage
3. Pneumothorax
4. Air embolism
5. Death

THIS CXR SHOWS

Projection: PA film, technically adequate.

>2cm pneumothorax on the right. Persistent changes of emphysema in the upper zones.

CLINICAL INTERPRETATION

CT guided lung biopsy carries a high risk of pneumothorax (between 30-50% in some series). Many are however, well tolerated and require no specific intervention to resolve.

Patients more likely to require intercostal drainage are patients with chronic lung disease (such as COPD) and patients with larger pneumothoraces.

Recognising small pneumothoraces can be difficult on CXR. Look at the apices in all chest films as this is where small pneumothoraces may hide. Look for the absence of normal lung markings (which can be more difficult in patients with emphysema who have reduced lung markings in any event) and look for a line, denoting the edge of the lung interfacing with the pleural air.

Q: Which of the following investigations will help diagnose this condition?

1. HRCT
2. Lateral plain CXR
3. Spirometry
4. CT chest and abdomen
5. Bronchoscopy

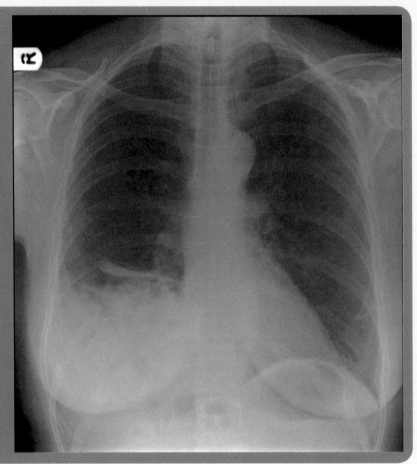

THIS CXR SHOWS

Projection: PA, well centred, adequate penetration, adequate field of view.

The heart, mediastinum and left lung are normal. The appearances suggest partial collapse of the right lower lobe. None of the right hemidiaphragm is clearly identified on the frontal projection and a lateral film may help clarify things further. An unusual pattern of density is projected in the lower zone area in the thorax with circular areas of gas density.

CLINICAL INTERPRETATION

This was an interesting case. CT confirmed right hemidiaphragm eventration containing loops of bowel (circular areas with gas density on the plain film) and an ectopic right kidney.

This is probably congenital as this lady gave no history of previous chest wall or abdominal trauma.

Surgical intervention with plication of the diaphragm can be offered and may benefit symptomatic individuals who show evidence of impaired static lung function and desaturation on exercise.

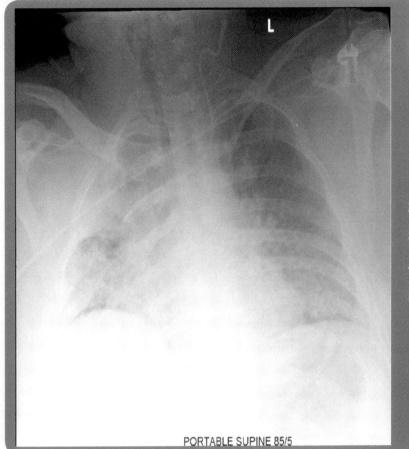

PORTABLE SUPINE 85/5

Q : What antibiotic would be most appropriate in this case?

1. Norfloxacin
2. Moxifloxacin
3. Levofloxacin
4. Ciprofloxacin
5. Co-amoxiclav

THIS CXR SHOWS

Projection: AP supine film. rotated

ECG electrodes visible. Left internal jugular vein CVP line in situ with tip lying in SVC.

Costophrenic angles difficult to visualise due to soft tissue shadowing. Opacification of the right lung field most dense in the right upper zone.

CLINICAL INTERPRETATION

This sort of film is very common in critical care. The patient has a right sided pneumonia on a background of ALD.

Patients with liver disease are at increased risk of infections including pneumonia. This is, in part, because many of the bodies primary immune defences are manufactured in the liver.

Patients with liver disease are also at high risk of mortality from pneumonia. Antibiotic treatment is the same as for patients without liver disease, with co-amoxiclav and clarithromycin recommended.

Q: Which of the following is **not** a complication associated with intravenous drug use?

1. *Pneumocystic Jirovecii pneumonia*

2. Empyema

3. Community acquired pneumonia

4. Cellulitis

5. Emphysema

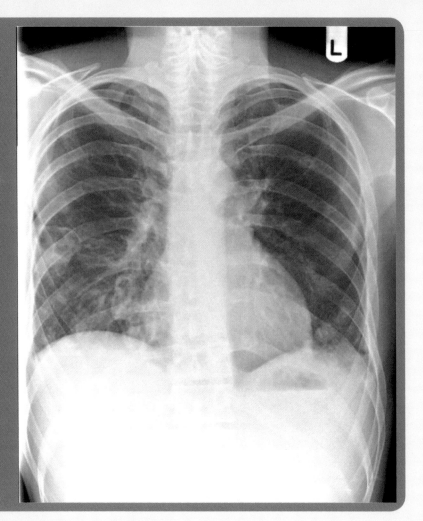

THIS CXR SHOWS

Projection: PA, technically adequate.

2cm opacity in the RMZ along with several other small round opacities throughout the lung fields.

CLINICAL INTERPRETATION

Patients with a history of intravenous drug misuse are at increased risk of deep vein thrombosis and pulmonary emboli, but are also at increased risk of soft tissue infections which may embolise. These "septic emboli" give the appearance seen in this chest x-ray.

Staphylococcus aureus is the most common organism.

IV drug misuse also predisposes to community acquired pneumonia and to empyema.

Emphysema is associated with cigarette and cannabis smoking but not with IV drug use.

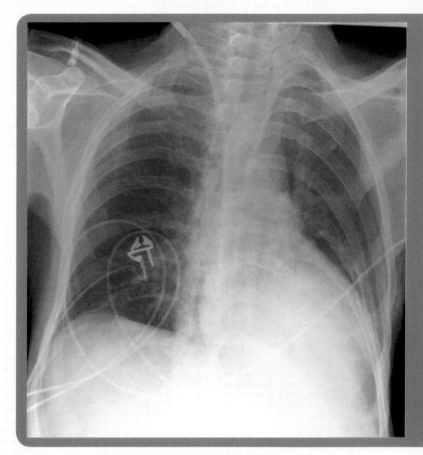

Q: What is the likely cause of the metabolic acidosis?

1. Community acquired pneumonia
2. Acute kidney injury
3. Salicylate overdose
4. Electrocution
5. Linezolid therapy

THIS CXR SHOWS

Projection: AP, rotated.

Left Costophrenic angle not possible to visualise.

Lung fields clear.

Right internal jugular vein triple lumen dialysis line in-situ.

CLINICAL INTERPRETATION

Metabolic acidosis is a feature of acute renal failure and this patient required dialysis.

Ideally these lines should lie at the level of the carina and so this line was pulled back several centimetres.

The classification of acute renal failure has recently been redefined. Patients should be assessed for acute kidney injury (AKI) using the RIFLE criteria[1] as

AKI stage 1- Creatinine 1.5x normal

AKI stage 2- Creatinine 2x normal

AKI stage 3- Creatinine 3x normal.

[1] *Crit* Care 2004, 8:R204-R212.

Q: Which of the following chest x-ray projections can be used to confirm pleural effusion?

1. Lateral decubitus
2. Lateral
3. Trendelenburg
4. Expiratory film
5. Supine

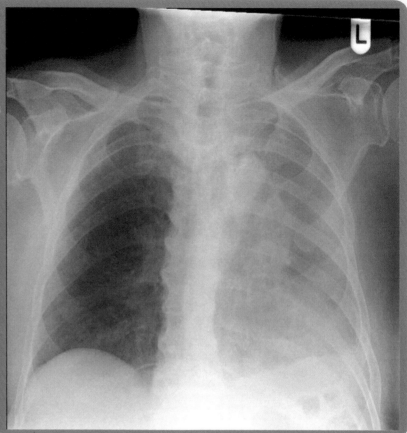

THIS CXR SHOWS

Projection: AP supine film, rotated

Opacification of the entire left lung field with ground glass appearance. Homogenous opacity at the left base consistent with pleural effusion. There is no mediastinal shift.

CLINICAL INTERPRETATION

This man had a left sided pleural effusion which was confirmed and aspirated under ultrasound guidance. The patient was lying in the supine position just prior to having the film taken. It is important to remember that although films are usually taken erect and therefore pleural effusions are usually in the dependent areas (i.e the lung bases) this is not always the case if the patient is supine.

Lateral decubitus films were used to detect small effusions before ultrasound became widely available.

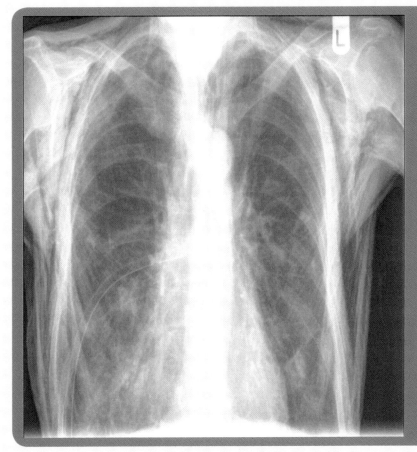

Q: Which of the following is not a recognised cause of surgical emphysema?

1. Dental surgery
2. Gun-shot wound
3. Blunt chest trauma
4. Pneumothorax
5. Endotracheal intubation

THIS CXR SHOWS

Projection: PA chest x-ray. rotated.

Severe surgical emphysema. Right intercostal chest drain.

The surgical emphysema gives the appearance of thin radiolucent areas throughout both lung fields but this is due to surgical emphysema in the overlying soft tissue.

CLINICAL INTERPRETATION

Surgical emphysema is a relatively common complication of intercostal chest drain insertion.

Usually it is a cosmetic problem rather than a serious medical issue and does not require treatment. In exceptional cases like this one, the swelling can be so severe as to compromise the patients airway. This patient required intubation.

It is important to check that the chest drain is properly sited as if the drain holes lie in the soft tissue this may contribute to the surgical emphysema. (this is not the case here)

Q : The following could be responsible for this appearance?

1. Sarcoidosis
2. Tuberculosis
3. Calcified lymph node
4. Carcinoid syndrome
5. Foreign body aspiration

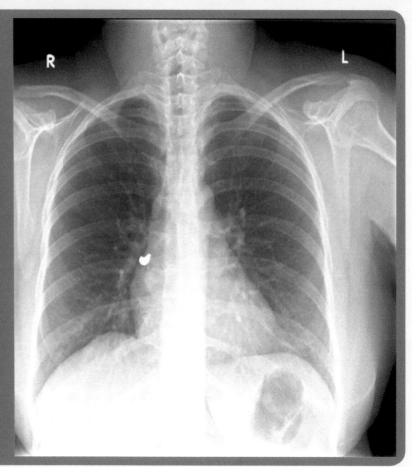

THIS CXR SHOWS

Projection: PA chest x-ray. rotated.

There is a radiolucent object in the RMZ consistent with an inhaled foreign body.

CLINICAL INTERPRETATION

This gentleman had aspirated a tooth into the right bronchus intermedius. Most foreign objects can be removed by using instruments introduced through the fibre-optic bronchoscope.

Natural reflexes prevent aspiration under normal circumstances and most patients experiencing aspiration have identifiable risk factors such as neurological disease (stroke, bulbar palsy), oesophageal pathology (causes of dysphagia) and impaired consciousness (alcohol and drug misuse and seizures).

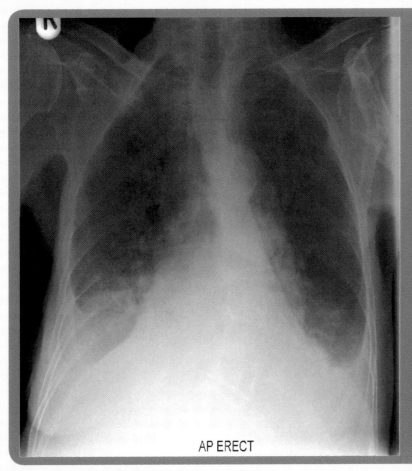

Q: Malignancy is associated with a transudate pleural effusion in:

1. <5%
2. 20%
3. 30%
4. 40%
5. 50%

AP ERECT

THIS CXR SHOWS

Projection: AP erect. Rotated to the right

Absent left breast shadow

Marked kyphoscoliosis

Cardiomegaly, even allowing for projection.

Bibasal homogenous shadowing consistent with bilateral pleural effusions.

CLINICAL INTERPRETATION

This appearance is not uncommon in clinical practice. Bilateral pleural effusions in association with cardiomegaly suggests heart failure, but the previous mastectomy, may point to recurrence of breast malignancy. The effusions should be aspirated to determine whether they are transudative or exudative and sent for cytological examination, microscopy and culture. Correlation with clinical presentation is, as always, essential; and a better quality CXR will usually give useful information.

<5% of transudate pleural effusions are due to malignancy

Q: What proportion of lung carcinomas occur in non-smokers?

1. 0%
2. 2%
3. 4%
4. 10%
5. 33%

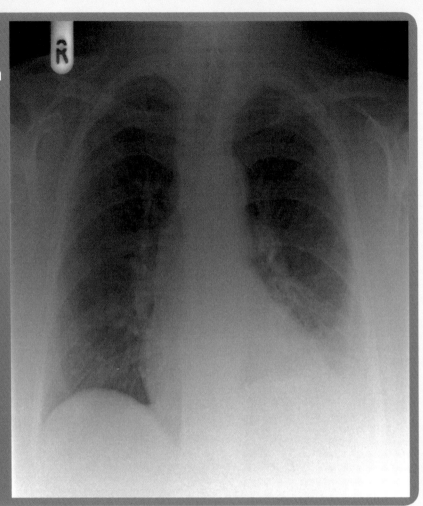

THIS CXR SHOWS

Projection: PA film.

Increased cardiothoracic ratio.

Left costophrenic angle obliterated by pleural effusion. Left basal homogenous shadowing consistent with pleural effusion.

CLINICAL INTERPRETATION

The constellation of symptoms of weight loss, a pleural effusion and breathlessness are suggestive of malignancy: up to 10 % of lung cancers occur in lifelong non-smokers. However, the differential includes pneumonia and empyema, both readily treatable. Lateral CXR and pleural ultrasound will help to differentiate between consolidation and effusion. The effusion should be aspirated and analysed to exclude infection and malignancy.

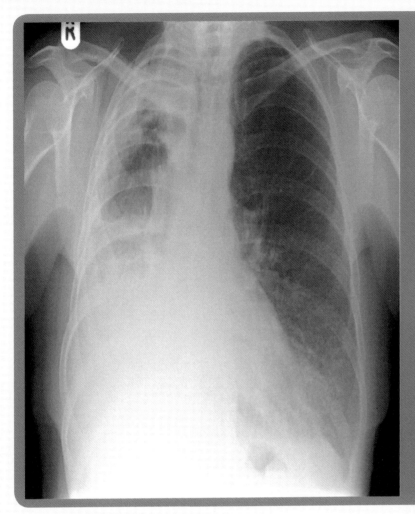

Q : The following is not present on this chest x-ray?

1. Dislocated right humerus
2. Pleural effusion
3. Tracheal deviation
4. Lung collapse
5. Right upper lobe consolidation

THIS CXR SHOWS

Projection: PA film, underpenetrated

There is loss of volume of the right lung with deviation of the trachea to the right.

There is patchy opacification involving the RUZ, and denser, more homogenous opacification occupying the lower half of the right hemithorax

CLINICAL INTERPRETATION

The differential here is between consolidation, collapse and effusion. The loss of volume, and tracheal deviation favour collapse, however trans-thoracic ultrasound is a simple, non-invasive test to confirm or refute the presence of pleural fluid, and should be carried out prior to the insertion of any intercostal drain if effusion is suspected. The collapse on this CXR is strongly suggestive of proximal obstructive lesion, and staging CT scan is indicated.

★★

Q : The x-ray shows

1. RUL collapse
2. Right hilar mass
3. RLL collapse
4. Right upper mediastinal mass
5. Left apical pneumothorax

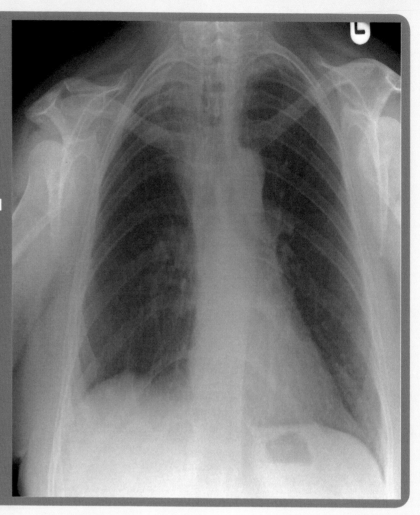

THIS CXR SHOWS

Projection: PA film, technically adequate

There is evidence of right upper lobe collapse with tethering of the right hemidiaphragm and streaky opacification of the right base. There is widening of the upper mediastinum. Blunting of the right costophrenic angle may indicate small pleural effusion.

CLINICAL INTERPRETATION

This film shows characteristic changes of right upper lobe volume loss with elevation of the horizontal fissure and a triangular opacity in the right upper zone. The right hemidiaphragm is elevated, and there is volume loss. This patient had a RUL lobectomy. In lung cancer this is carried out with curative intent, but is only truly curative in 50 % of cases. The widening of the mediastinum seen in this film may be recurrence, and staging CT scan of the thorax is indicated.

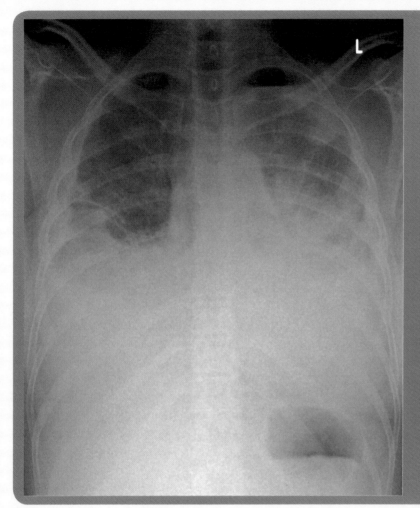

Q: The chest x-ray shows

1. Ring shadows

2. Lytic bone metastases

3. Malpositioned central venous line

4. Right apical pneumothorax

5. Coarse reticular opacification

THIS CXR SHOWS

Projection: PA film, technically adequate

There are large bilateral pleural effusions. There is interstitial opacitication in both midzones.

CLINICAL INTERPRETATION

Lymphangitis carcinomatosis (LC) is caused by malignant infiltration and invasion of pulmonary lymphatic channels. The lungs are a common site of metastases. Metastases are usually nodular but a significant minority are interstitial.

The most common primary sites are lungs, breast (as in this case), stomach and colon. Patients usually present with breathlessness and HRCT is the best imaging modality as appearance on plain chest x-ray can be similar to pulmonary oedema.

Q : What feature is **not** present on this chest x-ray:

1. Calcified granulomas
2. Hyperinflation
3. Prominent pulmonary vessels
4. Apical Pneumothorax
5. Apical Bulla

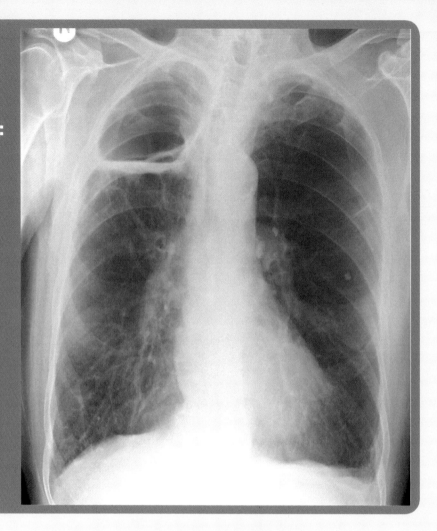

THIS CXR SHOWS

Projection: PA film. Technically adequate

Scoliosis, convex to the right

There is a large, thick-walled, right apical bulla. There are decreased lung markings in the upper zones consistent with emphysema. Pulmonary vascular prominence bilaterally. Features are consistent with chronic obstructive lung disease. Scattered calcified granulomas bilaterally.

CLINICAL INTERPRETATION

There are multiple abnormalities on this CXR, all of which are chronic. The right apical bulla is longstanding the thickened wall inferiorly could be mistaken for the wall of an abscess, but there is no air-fluid level. Calcified nodules on a CXR are usually a chronic change, usually of previous mycobacterial infection, or chronic granulomatous disease. Lung tumours do not calcify. Pulmonary congestion must be long standing before significant enlargement of pulmonary vessels occurs.

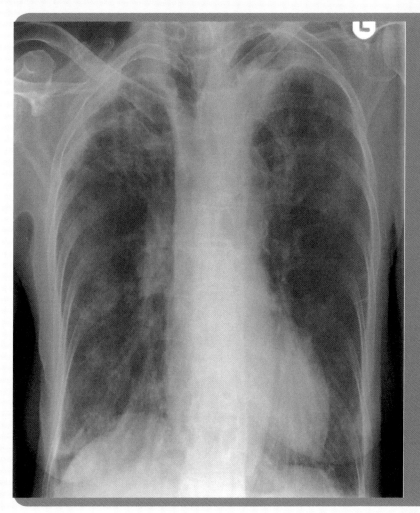

Q: Which of the following makes **TB less likely**

1. Apical opacification
2. Absence of cavitation
3. Bilateral opacification
4. Calcified pleural thickening
5. Granulomas

THIS CXR SHOWS

Projection: PA film, rotated.

There is a right hilar mass. The heart is of normal size, the lungs are hyper-inflated. The upper lobes show old changes of TB. There is a cavity, with an air fluid level in the LUZ. Widespread soft tissue infiltrates are seen throughout both lung fields.

CLINICAL INTERPRETATION

The differential for a cavity with air fluid level is:

- TB;
- abscess;
- squamous cell carcinoma;
- aspergilloma;
- hydatid cyst.

Associated mediastinal lymphadenopathy could be due to either infection, or malignancy. In this case the bilateral changes of previous TB show pre-existing cavity formation, which predisposes to secondary infection. Staging CT scanning of the thorax and bronchoscopy with targeted sampling are indicated.

Q: Immediate treatment should include all **except:**

1. Oxygen

2. Corticosteroids

3. Intravenous antibiotics

4. Central venous pressure monitoring

5. Vasopressors

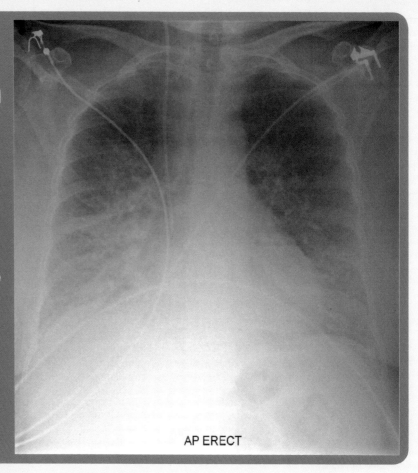

AP ERECT

THIS CXR SHOWS

Projection: AP erect film.

There is an intra-jugular central venous catheter with the tip in the right atrium. There is patchy, dense airspace opacification occupying both MZ and LZs, with air bronchograms most notable in the right lower zone. There is upper zone interstitial pattern showing.

CLINICAL INTERPRETATION

Airspace opacification, with air bronchograms, is pathognomic of a pneumonic process. This patient has Severe sepsis (defined as sepsis criteria with organ dysfunction- in this case respiratory failure) and septic shock (defined as hypotension not responding to adequate fluid resuscitation. Key measures in the Initial management of sepsis are

1. Early appropriate antibiotic therapy

2. Intravenous fluid resuscitation to mean arterial pressure > 65mmHg

3. Central venous pressure monitoring

4. IV insulin to maintain blood glucose <8.4mmol/l

5. Vasopressors and renal replacement therapy where required.

Surviving Sepsis Campaign: International guidelines for management of severe sepsis and septic shock: 2008 *Crit* Care Med 2008; 36:1394-1396

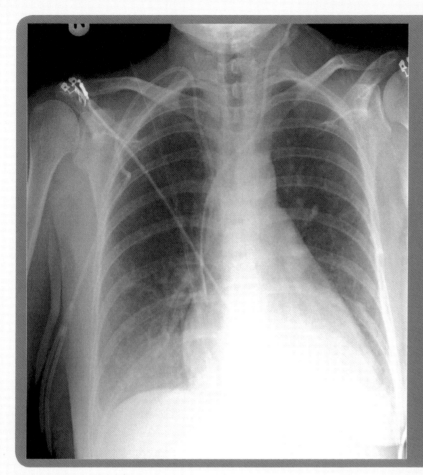

Q: What is the most likely diagnosis?

1. Ventilator associated pneumonia

2. Fungal pneumonia

3. Hospital acquired pneumonia

4. Community acquired pneumonia

5. Chicken-pox pneumonitis

THIS CXR SHOWS

Projection: PA film, technically adequate.

ECG electrodes visible. There is a right internal jugular tunnelled line, and a left internal jugular central venous catheter.

There is homogenous airspace opacification in the right lower zone, with air bronchograms

CLINICAL INTERPRETATION

Hospital acquired pneumonia is defined as pneumonia developing in patients who have been in hospital for more than 48 hours. During the first few days of hospital admission the nasal commensal bacteria brought in from the community are altered, giving a very different spectrum of causative pathogen. Common causes of hospital acquired pneumonia include *staphylococcus aureus* (often methicillin resistant); *pseudomonas aeruginosa*; *klebsiella species*; and *enterobacter species*. Antibiotic choices should be tailored to the likely causative organisms, particularly coverage of gram negative pathogens.

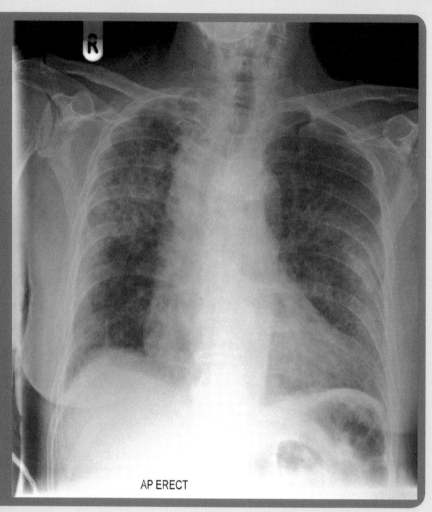

Q : Which of the following features of heart failure is present?

1. Bilateral mid-zone opacification

2. Upper lobe venous diversion

3. Kerley B Lines

4. Kerley A Lines

5. Bilateral pleural effusions

AP ERECT

THIS CXR SHOWS

Projection: AP film, over penetrated and rotated to the left.

Increased cardiothoracic ratio (but AP film). There is bilateral air space opacification extending to the peripheries, with bronchial wall thickening, and some interstitial change with an upper zone predominance. Notably there are no septal lines, upper lobe venous distension or pleural effusion present.

CLINICAL INTERPRETATION

This film shows no features of pulmonary oedema. The classical features of pulmonary oedema are: perihilar alveolar shadowing; upper lobe venous distension; cardiomegaly; Kerley B Lines; and transudate pleural effusions. The patient was initially treated as pulmonary oedema but in retrospect, another diagnosis seems more likely.

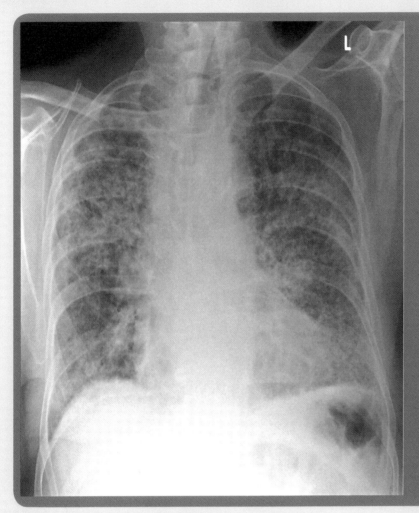

Q: Which of the following interstitial lung diseases may present in this way?

1. Non-specific interstitial pneumonitis (NSIP)

2. Acute interstitial pneumonitis (AIP)

3. Asbestosis

4. Sarcoidosis

5. Usual interstitial pneumonitis (UIP)

THIS CXR SHOWS

Projection: AP erect film.

There is rapid progression of the previously noted airspace opacification through all zones, bilaterally and peripheral interstitial changes. These appearances are may be due to acute interstitial pneumonia, pulmonary vasculitis, or rapidly progressive infection

CLINICAL INTERPRETATION

Acute Interstitial Pneumonitis (AIP) is a syndrome of rapidly progressive, acute lung injury of no known aetiology, resulting in Adult Respiratory Distress Syndrome (ARDS), and in 60 % of cases, death within 6 months; mean survival is 6 weeks. The CXR appearances are: airspace opacification due to leakage of proteinaceous fluid into the alveolar spaces; reticular shadowing and bronchial wall thickening due to interstitial oedema; normal cardiac shadow, if normal pre-morbidly; and no features to suggest left ventricular failure. Treatment is supportive, and speculative, at best.

Q : What symptom did he have which would explain this appearance?

1. Cough
2. Chest pain
3. Fever
4. Night sweats
5. Haemoptysis

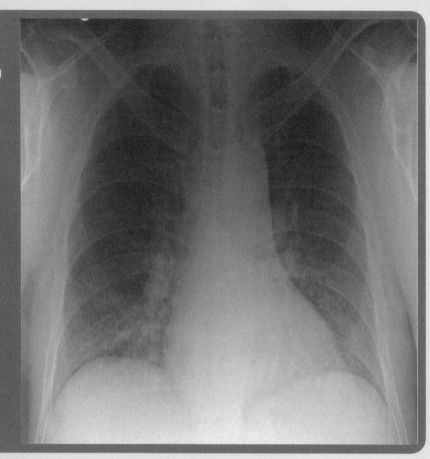

THIS CXR SHOWS

Projection: PA film technically adequate.

There is widespread reticulo-nodular shadowing, with a reticular predominance in the upper zones, and a nodular predominance in the lower zones.

CLINICAL INTERPRETATION

Such widespread nodular change is typical of miliary TB, and given his immunosuppressive regimen post transplant he is certainly at risk of mycobacterial infection. However, the differential of diffuse reticulo-nodular shadowing, particularly in an immunocompromised host includes: *Pneumocystis Jirovecii pneumonia*; lymphocytic interstitial pneumonia; Kaposi's sarcoma; toxoplasmosis; cytomagalovirus pneumonia; and miliary pneumonia. Established sarcoidosis can give rise to a similar appearance, but is not associated with immunosuppression.

This appearance was due to haemosiderosis, a long term complication following pulmonary haemorrhage

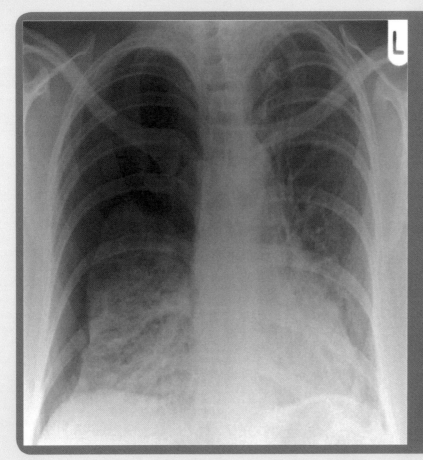

Q: What was the indication of this test?

1. Suspected TB
2. Bronchoalveolar cell carcinoma
3. Bronchiectasis
4. Lymphangioleiomyo-matosis
5. Interstitial Lung disease

THIS CXR SHOWS

Projection: PA film technically adequate.

There is a large right pneumothorax
There is background reticular/ nodular opacification throughout both lung fields.

CLINICAL INTERPRETATION

Spontaneous pneumothorax can be primary – in a patient with normal lung parenchyma – or secondary to pre-existing lung disease. This pneumothorax is iatrogenic, secondary to the biopsy. 5 – 10 % of patients undergoing trans-bronchial biopsy of the lung parenchyma will suffer pneumothorax,but only 20% of those will require chest drain insertion. This risk is increased in those with chronic lung disease, particularly empyhysema, and this group of patients are less likely to tolerate a pneumothorax. This makes the procedure, and the patient group, of high risk, and all patients should have a CXR 1 hour post intervention, or on developing new Symptoms.

Q: The diagnosis is:

1. Pulmonary oedema
2. Bilateral pneumonia
3. Usual interstitial pnumonitis (UIP)
4. Pulmonary arterial hypertension
5. Asthma

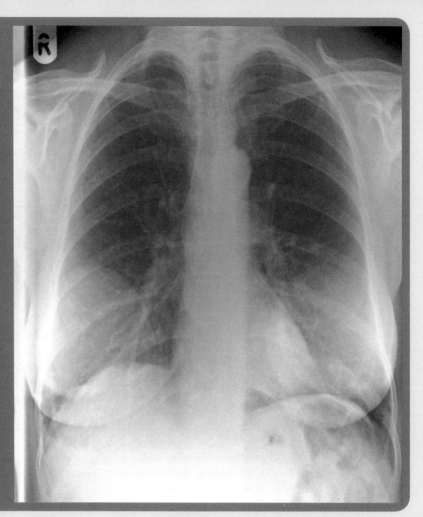

THIS CXR SHOWS

Projection: PA film. Technically adequate.

There is homogeneous opacification in both lower zones. The shadowing is rounded, and overlies both the hemi-diaphragmatic, and the cardiac silhouettes.

CLINICAL INTERPRETATION

This is the radiological appearance of breast implants. Increased shadowing in the lower zones due to breast tissue is obviously common in women, more so in young women, however, the homogenous shadowing, and sharp circular edges are not of physiological origin. Breast implants are seen in women of all ages and are inserted for a variety of reasons.

This 27 year old man has a testicular lump. This is his CXR

CXR 166

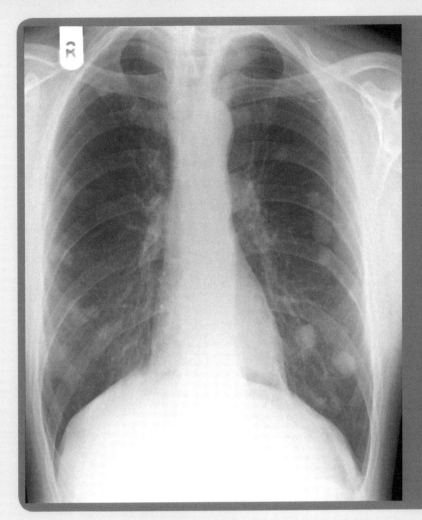

Q: What blood test may be elevated in this disorder?

1. Chorioembryonic antigen (CEA)

2. CA-125

3. CA19-9

4. Alpha feto-protein (AFP)

5. Alpha 1-antitrypsin

THIS CXR SHOWS

Projection: PA, well centred, well penetrated, adequate field of view.

There are multiple, bilateral, well circumscribed soft tissue shadows. The pulmonary vasculature is normal.

CLINICAL INTERPRETATION

Multiple pulmonary metastases. The most common cause of these so called "cannon-ball metastases" are renal cell carcinomas, however in younger males testicular tumours are an important differential. The differential of rounded lesions within the pulmonary parenchyma includes: primary bronchial carcinoma; carcinoid; hamartoma; lipoma. Multiple lesions as in this case, are invariably metastases.

In this case the diagnosis was a teratoma. These tumours are highly chemosensitive. Teratomas are associated with elevated AFP.

Q : Disorders that could predispose to this x-ray appearance in this man do **not** include:

1. Chronic thromboembolic pulmonary hypertension

2. Alcohol abuse

3. Cerebellar ataxia

4. Alpha-1-antitrypsin deficiency

5. Osteoporosis

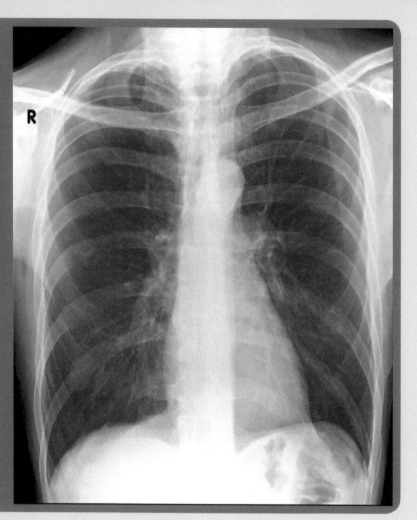

THIS CXR SHOWS

Projection: PA, well centred, well penetrated, adequate field of view.

Old fractures of the 8th, 9th and 10th ribs posteriorly.

Emphysematous changes bilaterally, with an upper zone preponderance.

CLINICAL INTERPRETATION

Rib fractures are a common finding on CXR, most are caused by a simple fall, or blunt trauma. Predisposing factors for multiple rib fractures of varying age are osteoporosis, instability and poor mobility. Patients with cerebellar ataxia are at particular risk of falls, and causes should be considered: alcohol, heavy metal poisoning, cerebellar infarction, space occupying lesion, multiple sclerosis.

There is no evidence of pulmonary infection to account for this man's COPD exacerbation. Non-pneumonic exacerbations of COPD are common, and are mostly viral in aetiology.

This 59 year old smoker is breathless, and has lost 1 stone in weight in the last month.

CXR 168

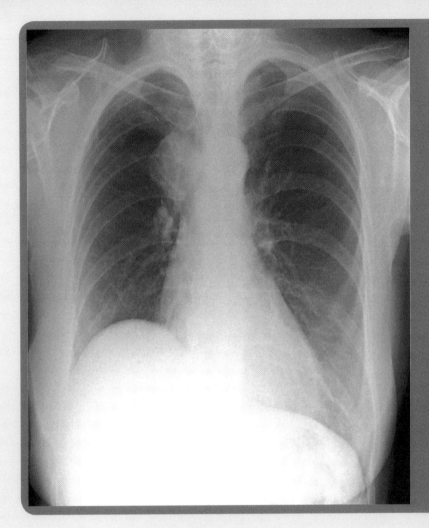

Q : The most likely diagnosis is?

1. Sarcoidosis

2. Lymphoma

3. Thymoma

4. Pulmonary embolism

5. Non small cell carcinoma

THIS CXR SHOWS

Projection: PA, well centred, well penetrated, adequate field of view.

The right hemi-diaphragm is markedly elevated. There is a soft tissue mass at the upper pole of the right hilum. The lung parenchyma are normal.

CLINICAL INTERPRETATION

This is a primary bronchial carcinoma with right phrenic nerve palsy, in turn causing elevation of the right hemi-diaphragm, The right hemi-diaphragm is usually higher than the left (to accommodate the liver) however a elevation of greater than 3cm is pathological. Causes of phrenic nerve palsy include: bronchial and mediastinal malignancy, most commonly; mononeuritis multiplex, previous phrenic nerve crush as treatment for TB, lobar collapse; partial lobar collapse following lung infarction; subphrenic abscess.

CXR 169

This 53 year old man presents with a history of haemoptysis, weight loss and night sweats. He is a student from Kazakhstan

Q: Which of the following management options would not be appropriate?:

1. Sputum analysis for Acid and Alcohol Fast Bacilli (AAFB)

2. Protective face masks for those involved in his care

3. Quadruple Therapy

4. Triple Therapy

5. Negative pressure isolation

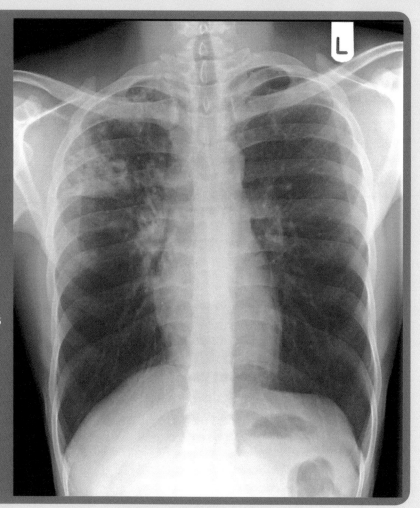

THIS CXR SHOWS

Projection: PA, well penetrated, adequate field of view.

There is consolidation with cavitation seen in the RUZ.

CLINICAL INTERPRETATION

This man had smear positive Tuberculosis (TB).

TB is transmitted by droplet spread. These may contain less than 10 bacilli.

Hospitalised patients must be placed in appropriate isolation. This includes a single room with negative pressure and adequate air exchanges. Persons entering the room must wear masks or respirators capable of filtering droplets from individuals suspected to carry multi-drug resistant TB. Quadruple therapy should be commenced empirically until fully sensitive TB is confirmed.

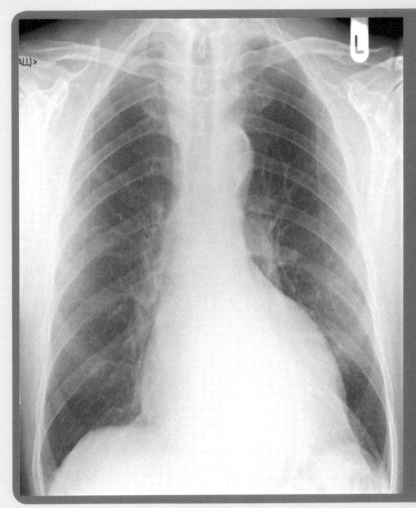

Q : Which of the following may predispose to this x-ray appearance?

1. Coxsackie virus
2. Cannabis abuse
3. Bronchial carcinoma
4. Osteoporosis
5. Asbestos exposure

THIS CXR SHOWS

Projection: PA, well centred, well penetrated, adequate field of view.

There is marked cardiomegaly.

The lung fields are clear.

CLINICAL INTERPRETATION

Plain radiology cannot assess cardiac function, and does not give an accurate measurement of cardiac size. However, a heart of this size, in a man of this age, on a PA CXR is clearly enlarged, and further investigation is warranted, usually with echocardiography.

There is no evidence of pulmonary oedema to explain this man's breathlessness

Q : The most likely diagnosis is:

1. Pulmonary embolism
2. Mitral stenosis
3. Bronchiectasis
4. Lung carcinoma
5. Tuberculosis

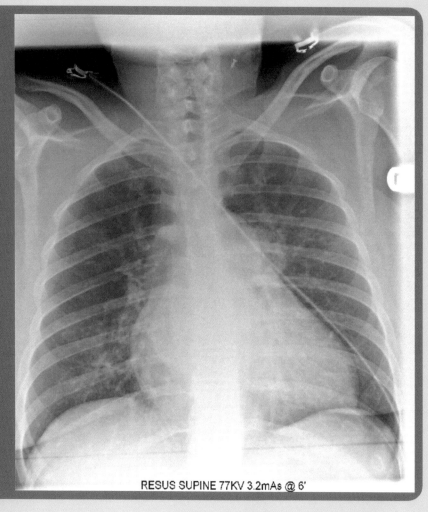

RESUS SUPINE 77KV 3.2mAs @ 6'

THIS CXR SHOWS

Projection: AP supine, well centred, well penetrated, adequate field of view.

Even allowing for the projection the heart size appears enlarged with an apparent double right heart border implying atrial enlargement. No focal collapse or consolidation is seen. Free intraperitoneal air cannot be excluded on a supine chest film. No acute bony injury detected.

CLINICAL INTERPRETATION

This woman had massive haemoptysis secondary to mitral valve disease leading to severe pulmonary venous hypertension.

Massive haemoptysis is defined as 100-600mls of fresh blood in a 24 hour period. Common causes are pulmonary embolism, lung carcinoma, bronchiectasis and cavitating infection. Non pulmonary causes are less common and not always easy to diagnose. In this case the plain film showed atrial enlargement and the diagnosis of severe mitral valve disease was confirmed on echocardiography. This woman had a history of rheumatic fever.

A 34 year old woman with previous empyema. Afebrile. Presents with left chest discomfort for several months.

CXR 172

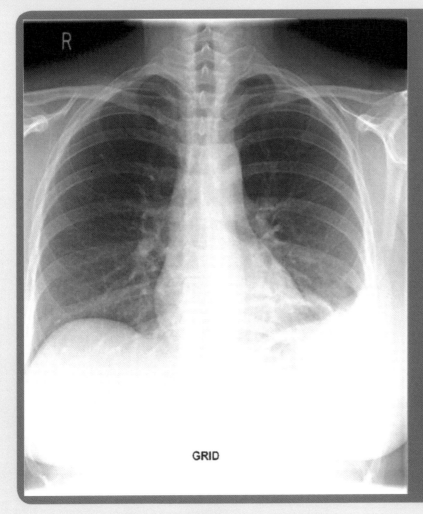

R

GRID

Q: Possible causes of this appearance do **not** include:

1. Hypoalbuminaemia
2. Pleural thickening
3. Elevated left hemi-diaphragm
4. Left empyema
5. Left haemothorax

THIS CXR SHOWS

Projection: PA film, technically adequate

There is homogenous left lower zone shadowing tracking up the pleural surface consistent with a pleural effusion.

CLINICAL INTERPRETATION

First impression would be left sided pleural effusion. However, the lateral plain film (next image) confirms pleural thickening. Decubitus films and chest ultrasonography would be alternative ways of confirming/refuting pleural effusion.

These two investigative methods are helpful as not only they would help with the diagnostic process but also prevent us from performing unnecessary diagnostic pleural aspiration.

Patients with previous empyema who have undergone chest drainage often have residual pleural thickening.

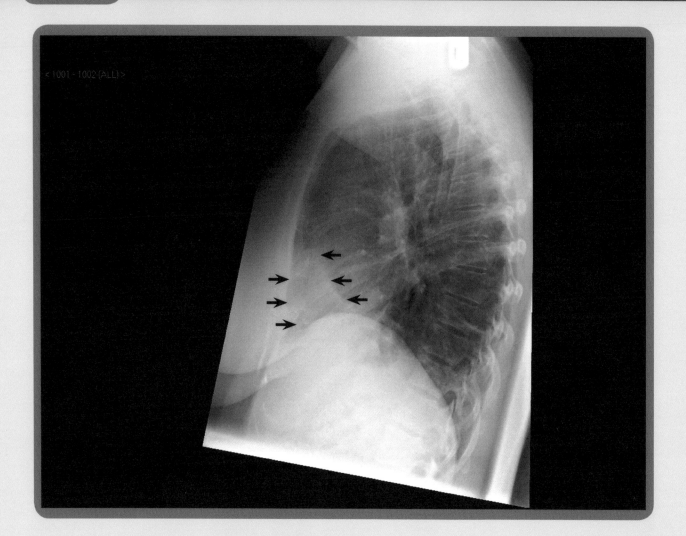

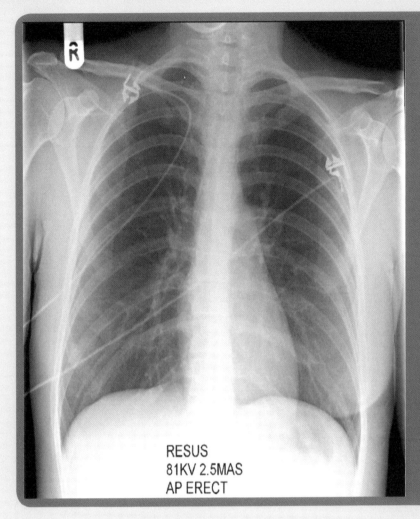

RESUS
81KV 2.5MAS
AP ERECT

Q: The most likely cause of her breathlessness is:

1. Right lower lobe pneumonia

2. Atrial fibrillation

3. Pulmonary embolism

4. Metabolic acidosis

5. Asthma exacerbation

THIS CXR SHOWS

Projection: AP erect film.

Normal chest x-ray

CLINICAL INTERPRETATION

The x-ray is normal.

Patients with DKA often have pyrexia and raised neutrophil count in the absence of infection.

It is inappropriate to treat patients with antibiotics purely on the basis of a raised white blood cell count or raised C-Reactive protein.

Nevertheless, infection is one of the potential triggers to diabetic ketoacidosis and appropriate microbiology samples (urine and blood cultures) should be obtained.

Metabolic acidosis is compensated by hyperventilation.

Q: Which of the following features are present on this chest x-ray?

1. Right lung tumour
2. Left lung tumour
3. Mastectomy
4. Bone Fracture
5. Hiatus hernia

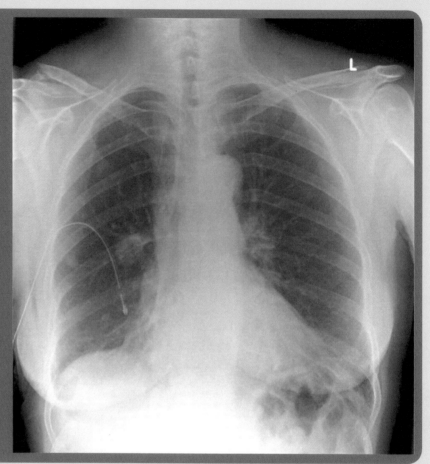

THIS CXR SHOWS

Projection: PA film, technically adequate

Fractured right clavicle.

There is a right intercostal drain in-situ. There is the appearance of a rounded mass at the right hilum which is most likely vascular.

CLINICAL INTERPRETATION

This is a case of a traumatic pneumothorax following fractured clavicle requiring an intercostal drain. With the other abnormalities on this x-ray it would be easy to miss the fractured clavicle.

Always complete a systematic evaluation of the plain film and don't get distracted by an obvious abnormality.

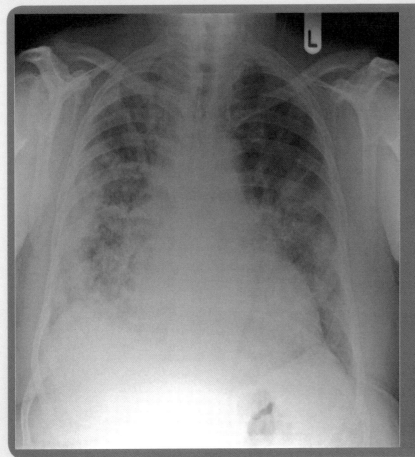

Q: Which of the following issues do you have to consider at presentation?

1. Anti-viral therapy

2. HIV test

3. Penicilin resistance

4. Negative pressure isolation facilities

5. Bronchoscopy

THIS CXR SHOWS

Projection: PA film, underpenetrated

Bilateral alveolar opacification consistent with multilobar pneumonia.

Cardiomegaly.

CLINICAL INTERPRETATION

Pneumonia secondary to *Legionella Pneumophilia*, a relatively common cause of community acquired pneumonia in Spain. Transmission occurs by means of aerosolization or aspiration of contaminated water. Cooling towers, respiratory therapy equipment and portable water distribution systems such as showers.

Extrapulmonary manifestations are common. These Include

- Hyponatraemia
- Diarrhoea and abdominal discomfort
- Hepatitis
- Myocarditis/Pericarditis
- Encephalopathy

Empirical treatment in this case would require a quinolone as *legionella* is not susceptible to Penicillin and a large percentage of *pneumococci* from Spain are penicillin resistant.

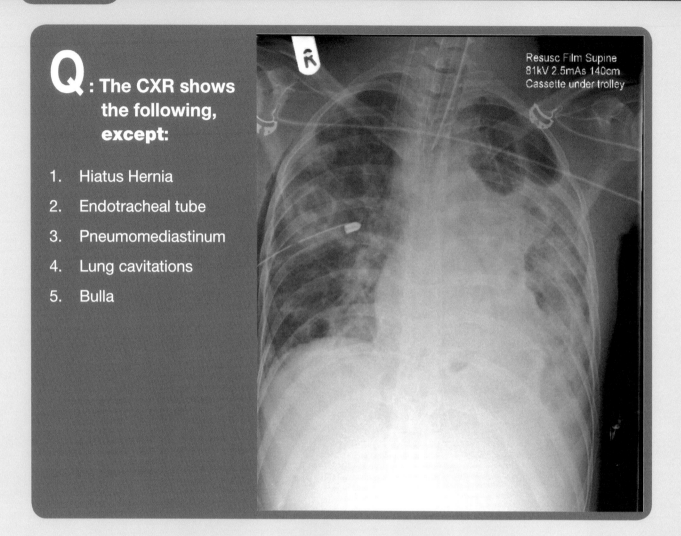

Q: The CXR shows the following, except:

1. Hiatus Hernia
2. Endotracheal tube
3. Pneumomediastinum
4. Lung cavitations
5. Bulla

Resusc Film Supine
81kV 2.5mAs 140cm
Cassette under trolley

THIS CXR SHOWS

Projection: Supine AP film, technically adequate

There is a right sided chest drain inserted with lung reinflation and subcutaneous emphysema. The air in the left apex persists and is confirmed to be a bulla on CT. There are large cavities scattered through both lungs. Air line noted along the left heart border suggestive of pneumomedistinum. Endotracheal, internal jugular line and cardiac leads noted.

CLINICAL INTERPRETATION

This unfortunate young lady did not survive.

Drug misuse can lead to a number of acute and chronic serious medical sequelae and plain chest radiography often helps with identifying some of those complications.

Intravenous drug misuse can be associated with septic emboli, cavitating lung infection and infections related to acquired immunodeficiency syndrome.

Inhaled drug misuse such as cannabis can lead to emphysema and bullous disease.[1]

[1] Thorax. 2000; 55(4):340-2

70 years old male. Chronic breathlessness and fatigue

CXR 177

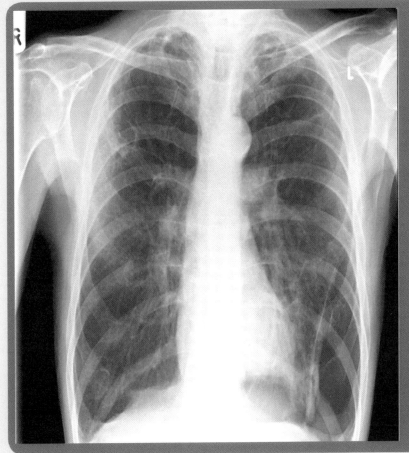

Q: What therapy is shown to improve mortality in this condition?

1. Long term oxygen therapy

2. Inhaled corticosteroid

3. Long term nebulised bronchodilators

4. Long term inhaled anti-cholinergic

5. Pulmonary rehabilitation

THIS CXR SHOWS

Projection: PA film. Technically adequate.

The lungs are hyperinflated with features of bullous lung disease. In the left lower zone there is a pneumothorax with a thick-wall surrounding it suggesting chronicity.

CLINICAL INTERPRETATION

This chest x-ray demonstrates the features and complications of severe emphysema.

The lung fields cover more than 8 posterior ribs. The ribs appear horizontal, the diaphragms appear flattened and the cardiac size appears relatively small. These are all characteristic features of hyperinflation.

Pneumothorax is a common complication of emphysema and bullous lung disease. Rupture of a bulla creates a significant air leak and these can be difficult to manage medically.

In COPD, only smoking cessation and long term oxygen have been shown to improve mortality.[1]

[1] MRC. Lancet 1981;i:681-6

Q: Which of the following procedures will obtain the diagnosis?

1. Bronchoscopy
2. Breast biopsy
3. Pleural biopsy
4. Thoracoscopy
5. Sputum for AAFB

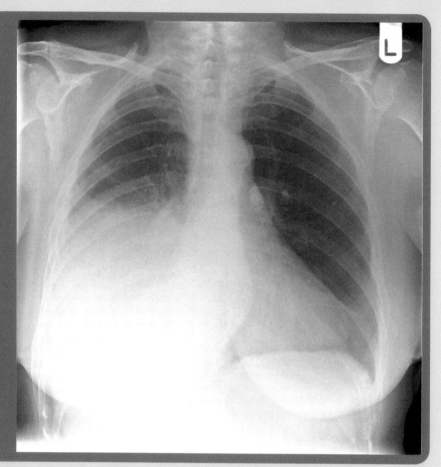

THIS CXR SHOWS

Projection: PA film. Technically adequate.

There is a large right pleural effusion. There is no associated pulmonary mass.

Calcified primary complex over left hilum.

CLINICAL INTERPRETATION

The combination of a right breast mass and a right pleural effusion suggests underlying metastatic breast carcinoma.

The diagnosis was confirmed by breast biopsy in this case.

In suspected malignant pleural effusion where there is no other obvious site to obtain a tissue diagnosis (such as a breast mass or enlarged lymph nodes) the diagnosis may be made by pleural fluid cytology. Blind pleural biopsy may also be used although this technique is now rarely performed due to its low sensitivity.

Medical thoracoscopy is increasingly the technique of choice in pleural effusions of unknown aetiology.

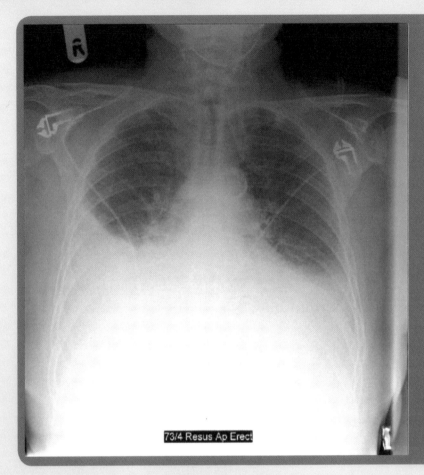

73/4 Resus Ap Erect

Q : Which of the following features does **not** usually accompany PND?

1. Orthopnoea
2. Ankle swelling
3. Sacral oedema
4. Wheeze
5. Pleurisy

THIS CXR SHOWS

Projection: AP erect film, under-penetrated

Cardiac silhouette appears enlarged even allowing for the projection.

Calcified aortic knuckle.

There are bilateral pleural effusions.

CLINICAL INTERPRETATION

The combination of bilateral pleural effusions and cardiomegaly in an elderly patient with paroxysmal nocturnal dyspnoea is clearly diagnostic of cardiac failure.

Paroxysmal nocturnal dyspnoea results from increased left ventricular filling pressure overnight. There is redistribution of fluid and increased renal retention of fluid promoting pulmonary oedema. The symptom has a high sensitivity for a diagnosis of heart failure.

If there is any diagnostic uncertainty the fluid should be sampled by thoracocentesis. It will be a transudate. By far the most common cause of bilateral transudates is left ventricular dysfunction, however hypoalbuminaemia, liver disease and constrictive pericarditis could give the same presentation.

Q: The most likely diagnosis is

1. Small cell carcinoma

2. Carcinoid syndrome

3. Squamous cell carcinoma

4. Broncho-alveolar cell carcinoma

5. Metastatic breast carcinoma

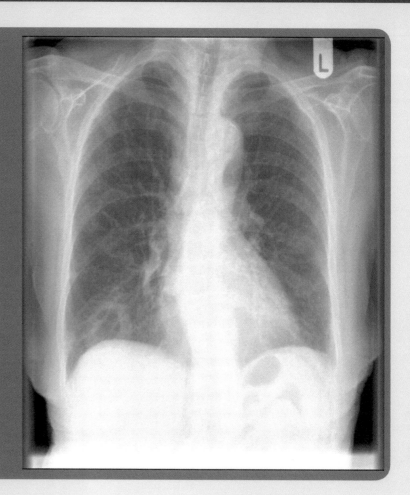

THIS CXR SHOWS

Projection: PA film, technically adequate.

Soft Tissues: Female, no abnormality.

Bones: no abnormality.

Cardiac Silhouette: normal

Pulmonary: there is a right lower zone cavitating lesion.

CLINICAL INTERPRETATION

Cavitating lesions have a wide differential including malignancy, tuberculosis, pulmonary abscess (*staphylococcal disease/Klebsiella pneumoniae*). In a 49 year old smoker with no symptoms of acute illness however, this strongly suggests a diagnosis of squamous carcinoma of the lung.

10% of squamous carcinomas cavitate. Squamous carcinoma is the most frequent cell type causing non-small cell carcinoma (NSCLC).

The diagnosis in this case was made by CT guided lung biopsy.

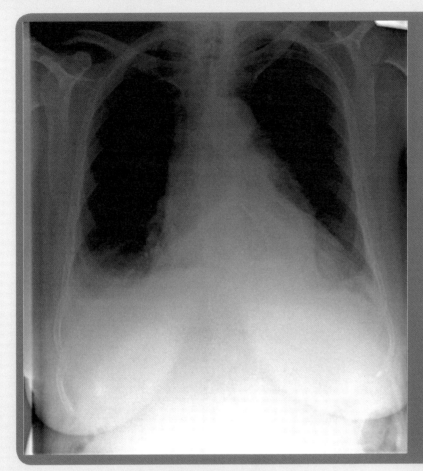

Q : This chest x-ray shows

1. Bilateral pleural effusions

2. Carotid artery atherosclerosis

3. Under-penetration

4. Coronary artery atherosclerosis

5. Gallstones

THIS CXR SHOWS

Projection: PA film, very over-penetrated

The cardiac silhouette appears enlarged. There is a fluid level behind the heart consistent with a hiatus hernia.

There are bilateral pleural effusions.

There is a nasogastric tube with the end probably in the fundus of the stomach.

CLINICAL INTERPRETATION

Enteral feeding was required for this lady following her stroke. The CXR was done to ensure appropriate

positioning of the nasogastric Tube. Penetrating the film makes it easier to visualise the nasogastric tube

Aspiration pneumonia is one of the leading causes of death after stroke. It is essential that all patients with a significant neurological deficit following stroke have a formal safety of swallowing assessment.

Patients failing a swallowing assessment will require to remain nil by mouth and may require enteral feeding to reduce the risk of aspiration.

Q: Appropriate management would include:

1. Intravenous diuretics

2. Revision of the right humerus prosthesis

3. Low molecular weight heparin (LMWH)

4. Pericardiocentesis

5. IV methyprednisolone

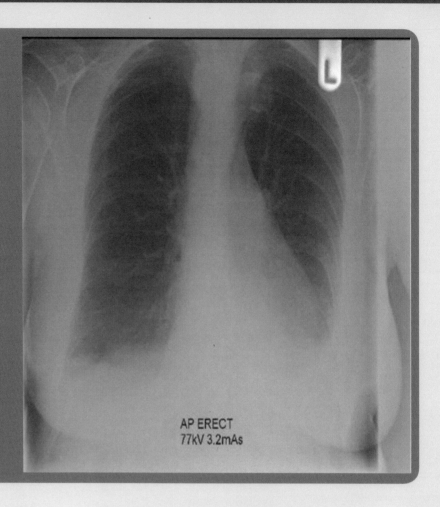

AP ERECT
77kV 3.2mAs

THIS CXR SHOWS

Projection: AP erect film. Underpenetrated. Inadequate field of view.

There are small bilateral pleural effusions larger on the left. There is a large opacity in the left upper zone which appears to be vascular.

CLINICAL INTERPRETATION

This patient has a pulmonary embolism (PE) post-operatively. Radiographic features of PE are extremely variable and clearly none are diagnostic. In the large PIOPED registry of PE the most common features were

- Enlarged pulmonary vessels 20%
- Normal 12%
- Oligaemia (Westermarks sign) 11%
- Hilar or mediastinal enlargement 7%

Atelectesis or parenchymal shadowing was common but was not significantly associated with PE.

Enlargement of the central pulmonary vessels as in this case is called the Fleischner sign. It is said to be indicative of PE, however in the PIOPED study, it was no more common in patients with confirmed PE than in patients without PE.

[1] Radiology 1993; 189(1):133-6

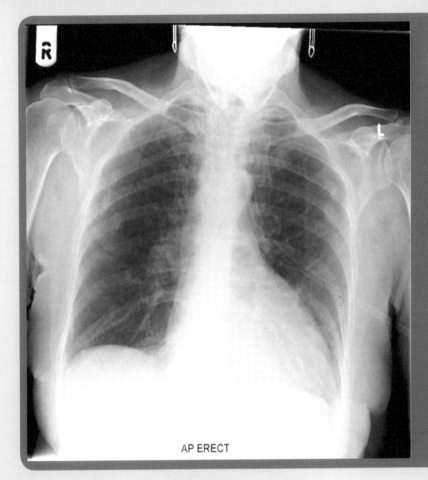

AP ERECT

Q : This patients management should include all of the following except......

1. Septic screen
2. Intravenous vitamins
3. Empirical antibiotics
4. Benzodiazepines
5. CT brain

THIS CXR SHOWS

Projection: AP erect film. Adequate field of view.

Ear-rings visible. Oxygen tubing visible. Bilateral healed rib fractures.

Increase in cardiothoracic ratio, but film is antero-posterior.

There is a generalised increase in bronchovascular markings but otherwise the lung fields are clear.

CLINICAL INTERPRETATION

This lady has radiographic features of alcohol abuse and smoking. The confusion was due to alcohol withdrawal.

Although not a perfect screening tool by any means, bilateral rib fractures of different ages are strongly associated with a history of alcohol abuse.

Alcohol abuse is also a risk factor for recurrent aspiration, aspiration pneumonia and community acquired pneumonia (particularly *Klebsiella species*).

Patients with a history of alcohol abuse are usually treated with benzodiazepines to prevent withdrawal and intravenous vitamins to prevent Wernicke-Korsakoffs syndrome.

Q: Which of the following is not a cause of type 2 respiratory failure?

1. Acute Asthma
2. Amyotrophic lateral sclerosis
3. Duchenne muscular dystrophy
4. Obesity
5. Opiate toxicity

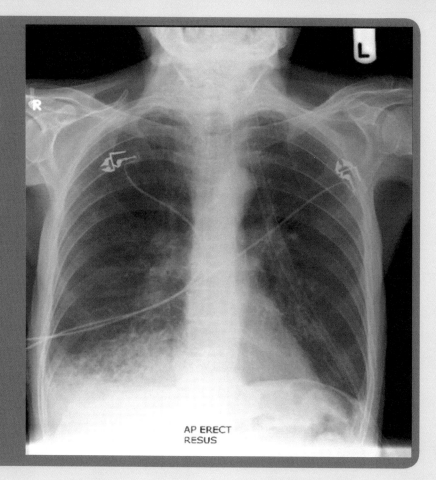

AP ERECT
RESUS

THIS CXR SHOWS

Projection: AP erect film. Technically adequate.

Oxygen tubing visible. ECG electrodes visible. There is consolidation in the right lower zone. There is a generalised increase in bronchovascular markings consistent with underlying COPD.

CLINICAL INTERPRETATION

This is a case of severe community acquired pneumonia in a patient with COPD.

Recent evidence suggests that the use of inhaled corticosteroids in COPD patients increases the risk of developing pneumonia[1,2]

Management of type 2 respiratory failure includes controlled oxygen therapy and bronchodilators. Non-invasive bi-level ventilation is required in patients not responding to standard therapy and may prevent intubation.

In asthma, a normal or raised pCO_2 is indicative of severe respiratory compromise and the need for invasive support. There is no role for bi-level ventilation in asthma.

[1] N Engl J Med. 2007: 22;356(8):775-89.

[2] Arch Intern Med. 2009: 9;169(3):219-29.

Answer: 1) Acute Asthma

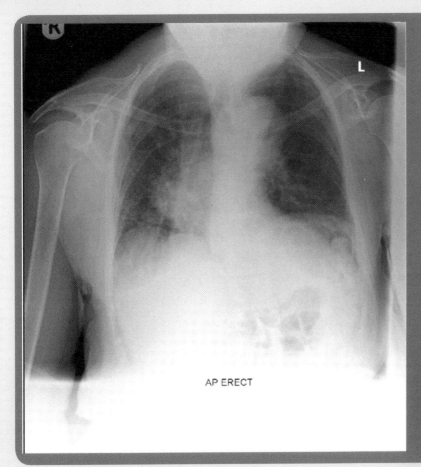

Q : This x-ray shows

1. Hiatus hernia
2. Right hilar mass
3. Peri-hilar "bat's wing" shadowing
4. Bochdaleks hernia
5. Fractured right clavicle

THIS CXR SHOWS

Projection: AP erect film. Underinspired, underpenetrated. Kyphosis make visualisation of the lung fields difficult.

The film is sub-optimal but there appears to be a mass adjacent to the right hilum.

In view of the rotation, a repeat plain film is recommended.

CLINICAL INTERPRETATION

This is a very poor quality x-ray. It is difficult to make the diagnosis of right bronchogenic carcinoma without a higher quality film.

To assess inspiration, we expect at least 6 anterior ribs or 10 posterior ribs to be visible within the lung field.

In an non-rotated film, the sternoclavicular joints should be equidistant from the midline.

The vertebrae are best used to assess the position of the midline.

Penetration is ideal if the vertebral bodies can be seen clearly behind the heart shadow

★ ★

Answer: 2) Right hilar mass

Q : Treatment failure in community acquired pneumonia may be due to all **except:**

1. COPD

2. Antibiotic resistant pathogens

3. Pulmonary embolism

4. Lung abscess

5. Empyema

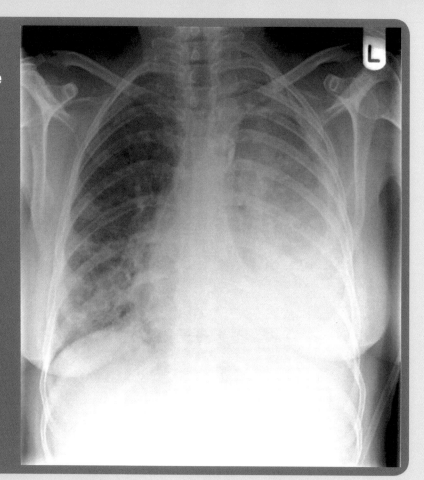

THIS CXR SHOWS

Projection: PA film. Technically adequate.

There is airspace opacification bilaterally in the lower zones. On the left there is a moderate pleural effusion.

CLINICAL INTERPRETATION

This is a case of community acquired pneumonia with parapneumonic effusion.

Parapneumonic effusions occur in 25-50% of cases of CAP. The majority are classified as simple parapneumonic effusions and resolve with appropriate treatment of the pneumonia. A complicated parapneumonic effusion is defined by a pleural fluid glucose < 2.2mmol/l, an LDH > 1000iu/L or a pH < 7.2 (Lights criteria). An effusion meeting these criteria requires a chest drain.

Empyema is defined as frank pus aspirated from the pleural space and intercostal drainage is mandatory.

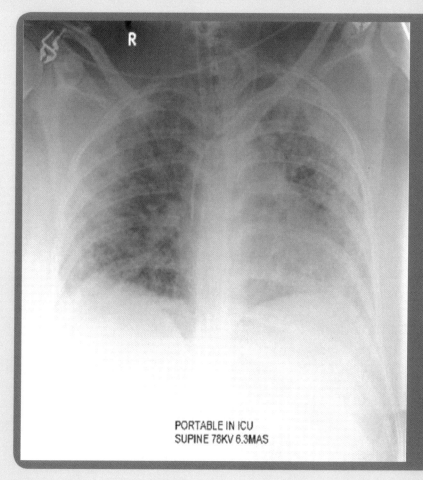

PORTABLE IN ICU
SUPINE 78KV 6.3MAS

Q: The chest x-ray shows:

1. Malpositioned ET tube

2. Adult Respiratory Distress Syndrome (ARDS)

3. Lymphocytic interstitial pneumonia (LIP)

4. Stage 4 Sarcoidosis

5. Hypersensitivity pneumonitis to interferon gamma.

THIS CXR SHOWS

Projection: AP supine film.

ECG electrodes visible.
left internal jugular central line.
There is gross airspace opacification bilaterally throughout all zones.

CLINICAL INTERPRETATION

The bilateral airspace opacification throughout the lung fields is typical of adult respiratory distress syndrome (ARDS).

ARDS is a clinical diagnosis rather than a radiological one. ARDS is defined as a PaO2/FiO2 ratio less than 200mmHg in the presence of a predisposing cause and bilateral alveolar infiltrates.. A ratio between 201 and 300mmHg is defined as acute lung injury (ALI).

A pulmonary artery wedge pressure <18mmHg is also a requirement, to differentiate the condition from left ventricular failure, which can also give this appearance.

Q: What is the diagnosis?

1. Hypertrophic obstructive cardiomyopathy

2. Brugada syndrome

3. Wolff-Parkinson White syndrome

4. Pulmonary embolism

5. Hypoplastic right heart syndrome

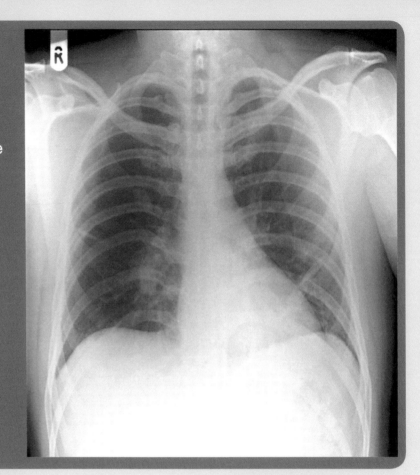

THIS CXR SHOWS

Projection: PA film. Technically adequate.

There are horizontal linear opacities in both mid-zones suggesting wedge shaped infarcts. There is general oligaemia particularly in the right lung field with prominent right pulmonary artery.

CLINICAL INTERPRETATION

No radiological features are considered useful for diagnosing pulmonary embolism and the diagnosis is based purely on clinical grounds.

In deciding whether to request further imaging, the British Thoracic Society recommend clinical probability assessment.

Patients are regarded as high risk if they have a risk factor for PE (e.g. immobility, malignancy, previous PTE) and PE is considered the most likely diagnosis. These patients require immediate imaging.

D-dimer assay is useful for patients at low to intermediate risk for PE (with only 1 of the above factors).

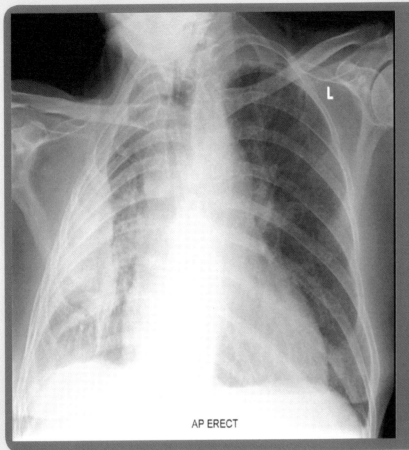

AP ERECT

Q: Possible causes of this appearance **do not** include

1. Asbestos exposure
2. Previous tuberculosis
3. Empyema
4. Hypercalcaemia
5. Pleurodesis

THIS CXR SHOWS

Projection: AP erect. Rotated.

It is difficult to assess tracheal position or mediastinal size due to rotation.

There is a large calcified pleural plaque on the right with evidence of significant volume loss.

CLINICAL INTERPRETATION

This x-ray shows the consequences of a previous empyema. This gentleman presented with primary empyema a year previously and failed to improve despite chest drainage and thoracoscopic surgery. Pleural aspiration revealed *streptococcus milleri*. This is currently the most frequent organism isolated from empyema in the UK.[1,2]

Chronic pleural changes like these can lead to a restrictive ventilatory defect accounting for this gentleman's breathlessness.

[1] *N Engl J Med.* 2005;352:865-874.

[2] Throax doi:10.1136/thx.2008.105080

Q : What is the most likely cause of this?

1. Soft tissue shadowing

2. Pneumoperitoneum

3. Disseminated malignancy

4. Osteoporosis

5. Community acquired pneumonia

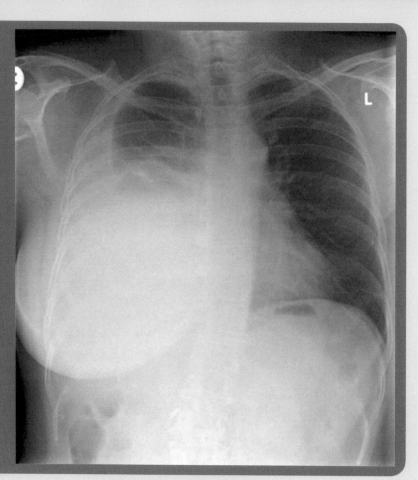

THIS CXR SHOWS

Projection: PA film, technically adequate.

Left mastectomy. homogenous opacification in the right lower zone consistent with a right pleural effusion.

CLINICAL INTERPRETATION

The diagnosis of metastatic breast carcinoma is strongly suggested by this radiograph showing a left mastectomy (due to previous breast carcinoma) and a large right sided pleural effusion.

Common sites of metastases for breast carcinoma are bones, liver, brain, lungs and the pleura as in this case.

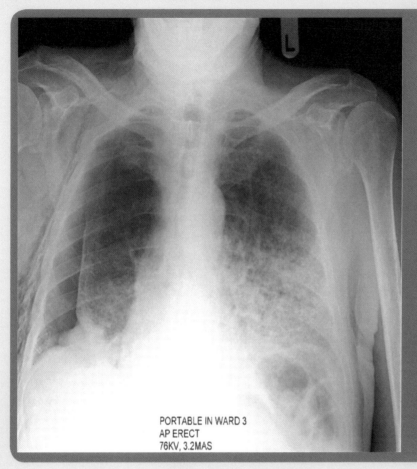

PORTABLE IN WARD 3
AP ERECT
76KV, 3.2MAS

Q: The chest x-ray shows the following except....

1. Bullous lung disease
2. Interstitial lung disease
3. Subcutaneous emphysema
4. Pneumothorax
5. Intercostal chest drain

THIS CXR SHOWS

Projection: AP erect film. Rotated. Underpenetrated.

Wide spread dense reticular nodular opacification throughout both lungs. Right pneumothorax with associated surgical emphysema. There is a small chest drain visible at the right costophrenic angle.

CLINICAL INTERPRETATION

Pneumothorax can complicate many chronic lung diseases.

Most frequently it complicates emphysema but also occurs

More frequently in patients with interstitial lung disease as in this case of idiopathic pulmonary fibrosis.

It is unlikely that a pneumothorax will resolve with simple tube drainage in a patient with such significant pulmonary parenchymal disease. In this case, the pleura is thickened suggesting a degree of chronicity making it less likely this will resolve.

CXR 192

A 71 year old lady with pneumonia failing to respond to antibiotics. She has a raised peripheral eosinophil count

Q: Which of the following is **not** associated with a raised peripheral eosinophil count:

1. Asthma

2. Allergic bronchopulmonary aspergillosis (ABPA)

3. Anti-fungal therapy

4. Hydatid cyst

5. Hydrocortisone

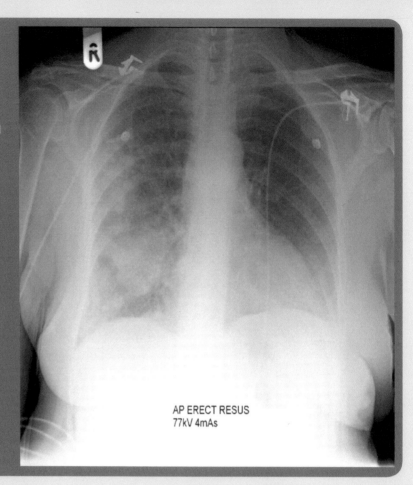

AP ERECT RESUS
77kV 4mAs

THIS CXR SHOWS

Projection: AP erect film. Technically adequate

Homogenous opacification in the right mid zone.

CLINICAL INTERPRETATION

This is a case of eosinophilic pneumonia and this diagnosis was confirmed by an elevated eosinophil count on bronchoalveolar lavage.

There is often no identifiable trigger to eosinophilic pneumonia although drugs, environmental toxins and parasite infections are associated with the diagnosis.

In patients with pneumonia not responding within 3-4 days to empirical antibiotics, an alternative diagnosis should be considered.

Eosinophilic pneumonia responds rapidly to steroid therapy.

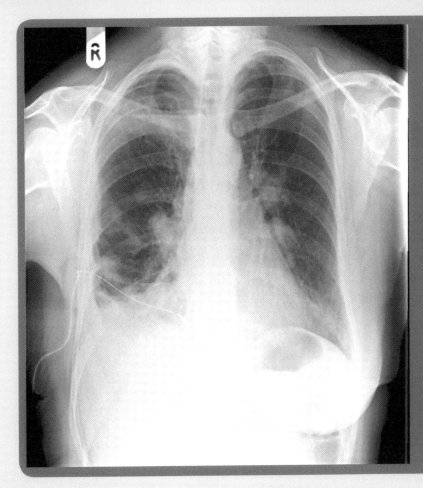

Q : The following may explain her confusion except:

1. Syndrome of innappropriate Anti-diuretic hormone (SIADH)

2. Brain metastases

3. Hypoxaemia

4. Intercostal drain

5. Opiate toxicity

THIS CXR SHOWS

Projection: PA film. Technically adequate.

Absent right breast shadow suggesting mastectomy. Right intercostal drain in situ.

Multiple rounded opacities suggestive of metastatic disease. Residual blunting of the right costophrenic angle suggesting small effusion.

CLINICAL INTERPRETATION

The radiological appearances are highly suggestive of metastatic breast carcinoma. The mastectomy suggests previous surgery for breast cancer and the lung and pleura are frequent sites of metastatic spread for this disease.

Given this clinical scenario the most likely cause of confusion is brain metastases. In reality, this lady had a sodium of 118mmol/l and subsequently had a diagnosis of syndrome of inappropriate ADH (SIADH).

Q: The following jobs can explain this CXR appearance, except?

1. Navy officer
2. Laboratory technician
3. Car mechanic
4. Jute mill worker
5. Plumber

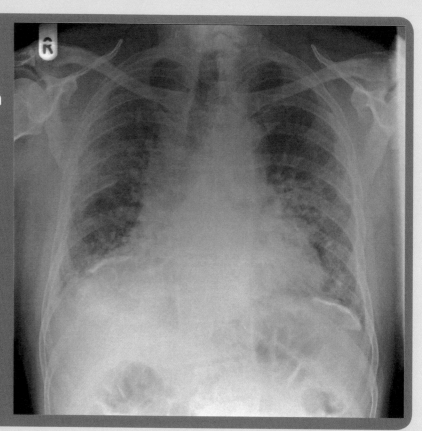

THIS CXR SHOWS

Projection: PA film. Technically adequate and central.

There is cardiomegaly and bilateral calcified pleural plaques. There is fibrotic change with small volume of the lungs. There is an air bronchogram seen in the LMZ peripheral hilar region suspicious of infection.

CLINICAL INTERPRETATION

This man has asbestos related lung disease and evidence of lower respiratory tract infection.

Asbestos is a naturally occurring silicate mineral with long, thin fibrous crystals. Asbestos became increasingly popular among builders and manufacturers in the late 19th century because of its resistance to heat, electricity and chemical damage. It also has useful tensile and insulating properties.

Many occupations have made use of asbestos fibres in their trade but also led to significant exposure and lung toxicity in their victims. Manifestations of lung toxicity occur a few decades later and it's essential that you obtain an accurate occupational history to aid successful compensation.

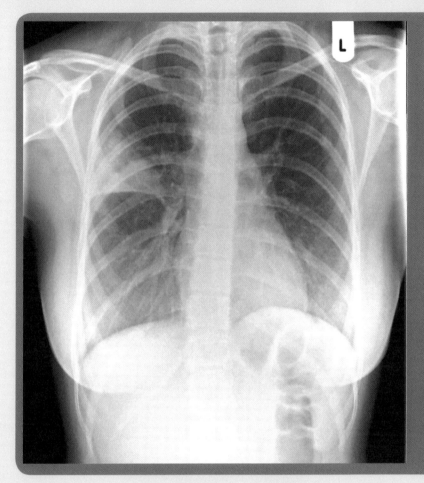

Q : Where is the abnormality?

1. Apical segment RUL
2. Anterior segment RUL
3. Posterior segment RUL
4. Superior segment RML
5. None of the above

THIS CXR SHOWS

Projection: PA film. Technically adequate.

There is alveolar shadowing in the right upper zone above the horizontal fissure.

CLINICAL INTERPRETATION

This is a case of community acquired pneumonia.

Pneumococcus is the commonest organism. Pneumonia frequently complicates chronic lung diseases and has recently been associated with the use of inhaled corticosteroids (the mainstay of treatment for asthma and COPD). It is clear from the chest x-ray that the consolidation is in the right upper lobe as it is clearly seen above the horizontal fissure. The right upper lobe is

divided into 3 segments- anterior, posterior and apical. If you want to be very clever you can say this consolidation lies in the anterior segment- as this segment lies adjacent to the horizontal fissure!

Answer: 2) Anterior segment of RUL

Q: The features of interstitial lung disease on chest x-ray frequently includes the following **except**:

1. Nodules
2. Reticular shadowing
3. Ground glass shadowing
4. Cavitation
5. Cardiomegaly

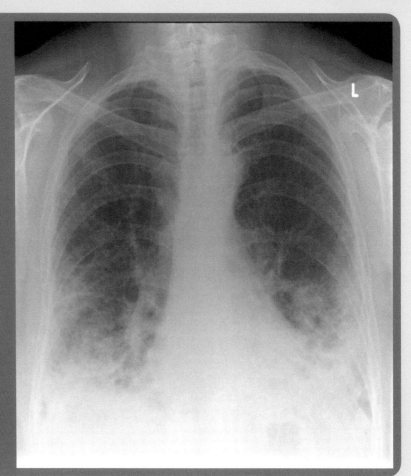

THIS CXR SHOWS

Projection: PA film. Underpenetrated.

Airspace shadowing in both lower zones.

CLINICAL INTERPRETATION

This lady underwent lung biopsy and the diagnosis of acute interstitial pneumonia was made. AIP is one of the interstitial lung diseases. It progresses over days or weeks and is synonymous with the "Hamman-Rich syndrome"

It is defined clinically as rapidly progressive respiratory failure in a patient with previously normal lungs.

High dose corticosteroids and cyclophosphamide are most commonly used but the condition is often fatal.

Answer: 5) Cardiomegaly

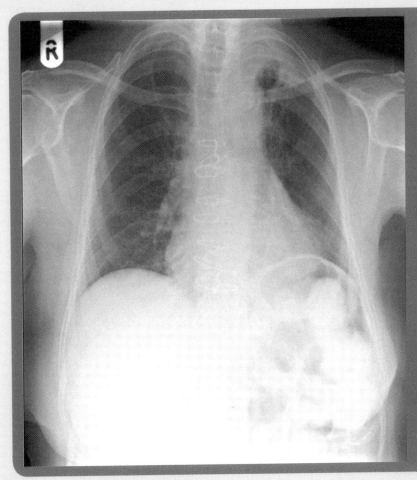

Q : Which of her medications could be responsible?:

1. Ethambutol
2. Ciprofloxacin
3. Isoniazid
4. Pyridoxine
5. Methotrexate

THIS CXR SHOWS

Projection: PA film. Technically adequate

Mid-line sternotomy sutures present.

There is loss of volume and scarring on the left upper lobe and left pleural thickening.

CLINICAL INTERPRETATION

Some manifestations of previous pulmonary Tuberculosis infection.

Pulmonary TB tends to affect the upper lobes and chronic infection led to pleural thickening volume loss and bronchiectasis. The consequences of tuberculosis infection and treatment in the pre-chemotherapy era are widespread in respiratory clinics across the country.

Optic neuritis is a rare complication of Ethambutol therapy.

Q: Which of the following has not been used in the treatment of tuberculosis?

1. Phrenic nerve surgery

2. Streptomycin

3. Artificial pneumothoraces

4. Plombage

5. Infliximab

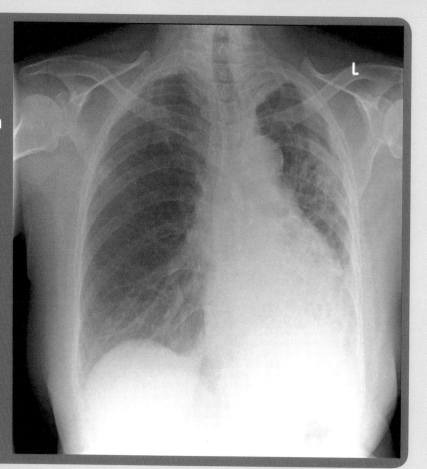

THIS CXR SHOWS

Projection: PA film. Technically adequate

There is left apical scarring. There is left pleural calcification and volume loss.

CLINICAL INTERPRETATION

This is old tuberculosis. The patient was tired due to anaemia and had no evidence of active tuberculosis.

Consequences of old TB are common throughout the world.

Common radiographic features are upper zone fibrosis, collapse and volume loss. Old calcified granulomas or lymph nodes are commonly seen. The patient in this case had a tuberculous empyema.

Treatments prior to the introduction of antibiotics may also be seen on the CXR. Thoracoplasty, lobectomy and phrenic nerve crush procedures were all commonly performed prior to the introduction of effective chemotherapy.

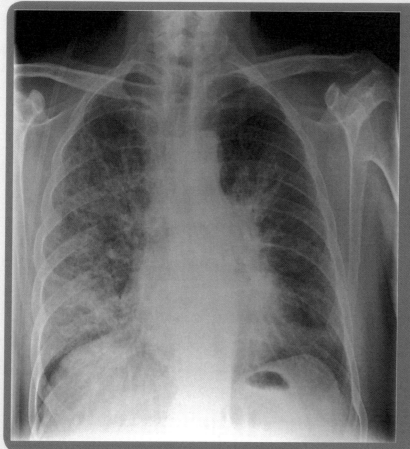

Q: Which of the following diagnoses is **not** commonly associated with this CXR appearance?

1. Miliary Tuberculosis

2. Hypersensitivity Pneumonitis (HP)

3. Sarcoid

4. Lymphangitis Carcinomatosis (LC)

5. Pulmonary Oedema

THIS CXR SHOWS

Projection: PA film. Technically adequate

There is diffuse, dense reticular opacification involving both lung fields but worse on the right in association with a left hilar mass.

CLINICAL INTERPRETATION

This is a case of Lymphangitis Carcinomatosis (LC).

In LC the accuracy of chest radiography is less than 25%.

The appearances are similar to those of interstitial pneumonias and pulmonary oedema. Pulmonary oedema tends to be more symmetrical in appearance than LC and interstitial pneumonias but the diagnosis is mainly derived from the patient's past history and response to treatment offered.

HRCT has higher sensitivity than plain films in detecting LC, but without relevant clinical features would still offer other differentials such as sarcoidosis, Kaposi sarcoma, lymphoma and hypersensitivity pneumonitis.

★ ★ ★

Answer: 1) Miliary Tuberculosis

A 72 year old man presents with tiredness, fever and is known to have a history of nasal ulceration, sinusitis and ocular disease

Q: Which of the following is the most likely diagnosis?

1. Mycobacteria Kansasii

2. Mycobacteria Bovis

3. Wegener's Granulomatosis (WG)

4. Mycobacterial Tuberculosis

5. Goodpasture's Syndrome

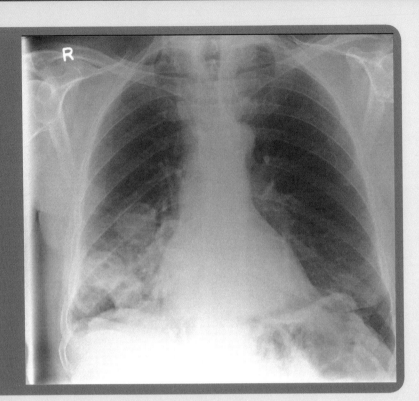

THIS CXR SHOWS

Projection: PA film. Under penetrated but otherwise technically adequate.

Four cavitating round lesions are present in the right chest. The walls of the cavities are quite thick. Blunting of the right costophrenic angle suggestive of a pleural effusion.

CLINICAL INTERPRETATION

The diagnosis of Wegener's Granulomatosis (WG) is suspected when patients present with sinusitis, nasal ulceration, other upper and lower respiratory tract symptoms such as cough, haemoptysis and breathlessness.

Renal involvement is usually detected at presentation by detecting blood and protein in the urine and constitutional symptoms such as fever and weight loss are also common. WG can also present neurologically, commonly with ocular manifestations but symptoms can be extremely varied; and include seizures, meningeal irritation and cranial neuropathies.

Routine laboratory tests are often non specific but may show raised markers of inflammation and anaemia is present in 50% of cases at presentation. c-ANCA assay is positive in more than 70% of cases but has a positive predictive value of only 50%.

APPENDIX

The Top to Bottom approach to CXR interpretation

1. Look for the most obvious abnormality first by examining the lung fields. Your eyes are going to be drawn here anyway, so there is no point fighting your natural instincts.- This is the "**Initial Review**". Once you have described the major abnormality in detail, move on systematically to the rest of the film.

2. We proceed "top to bottom". Examine the clavicles and shoulder joints. While you are looking at the **bony structures**, proceed to systematically examine the ribs for fractures.

3. Take a second, more systematic, look at the lung fields. Refer to the anatomy above as a reference. Look first at the right upper lung field and interface with the mediastinum- this is where to look for right upper lobe pathology. Look at the right heart border- this is where to look for right middle lobe pathology. Then examine the right hemidiaphragm. Any interruption of the hemidiaphragm suggests right lower lobe pathology. Then take a second look at the left upper lung field- this is where to look for left upper lobe pathology. Then look at the left heart border- any interruption of this border indicates lingula pathology. Then examine the left hemidiaphragm for lower lobe pathology. Finally, take a **second look** at the hilar shadows on both sides. Remember that the left hilum is slightly higher than the right because the left main pulmonary artery passes above the left main bronchus.

4. Examine the cardiac and mediastinal structures for abnormalities, including assessing the cardiothoracic ratio.

5. Look below the diaphragms carefully for pneumoperitoneum (air under the diaphragm) and for the gastric bubble.

6. Finally, take another look at the apices, behind the heart and diaphragms. This is where occult pathology is often missed.

INDEX

CPSIA information can be obtained
at www.ICGtesting.com
Printed in the USA
LVIC040838051012
3077LVUK00008B

* 9 7 8 1 9 0 5 0 0 6 3 6 6 *